Handbook of Trigeminal Neuralgia

Girija Prasad Rath
Editor

Handbook of Trigeminal Neuralgia

Springer

Editor
Girija Prasad Rath
Department of Neuroanaesthesiology and Critical Care
Neurosciences Centre
All India Institute of Medical Sciences
New Delhi
India

ISBN 978-981-13-2332-4 ISBN 978-981-13-2333-1 (eBook)
https://doi.org/10.1007/978-981-13-2333-1

This Springer imprint is published by the registered company Springer Nature Singapore Pte Ltd.
The registered company address is: 152 Beach Road, #21-01/04 Gateway East, Singapore 189721, Singapore

Dedicated to the loving memory of
my late mother, Smt. Indu Rath

Foreword

It gives me great pleasure and immense satisfaction to write the foreword for *Handbook of Trigeminal Neuralgia*, edited by Prof. Girija Prasad Rath of the All India Institute of Medical Sciences (AIIMS), New Delhi. The subject of trigeminal neuralgia is very close to my heart as I have been involved with the management of this painful affliction for almost four decades of my career. I established the practice of pain in the Neurosciences Centre of AIIMS where the editor, Prof. Rath, is currently working. It is heartening to see the Pain Clinic, which was established nearly two decades ago, continuing to cater to many patients of trigeminal neuralgia with latest treatment strategies. I give full credit to Prof. Rath for editing this excellent handbook apart from contributing a number of chapters himself; the book covers almost all the aspects of trigeminal neuralgia available in the literature. All the contributors have done full justice to the subject. There are descriptions of newer treatment options, such as injection of botulinum neurotoxin and neuromodulation, which may encourage practitioners to look for alternative options other than the usual conventional modalities. I will not hesitate to recommend this book to all medical professionals involved in the management of intractable pain of face and head.

Surinder Singh Saini
Neuroanaesthesia and Pain Management,
Paras Hospitals, Gurugram, Haryana, India

Former Head, Department of Neuroanaesthesia,
All India Institute of Medical Sciences, New Delhi, India

Preface

Trigeminal neuralgia is an extremely debilitating condition unlike many other medical ailments. The paroxysmal pain is so unbearable that it completely breaks down the mental strength of a person, sometimes to the point of driving him/her to even attempting suicide. I realised the enormity of this problem as a resident of Neuroanaesthesia at Neurosciences Centre of the All India Institute of Medical Sciences (AIIMS), New Delhi. It was very painful while attending to these patients in the pain clinic to listen to their stories of long-term suffering and console them during an occasional outburst of cry. My mentor, Prof. Parmod Kumar Bithal, could realise my growing interest in this particular group of patients. As a senior faculty and head of the department, Dr. Bithal gave me a lot of liberty to execute treatment plans with his constant encouragements. A lot of discussions with him further motivated me to participate regularly in treatment strategies for patients with trigeminal neuralgia, who were referred to us by colleagues from the specialities of neurology and neurosurgery. The intention to do something more for these patients fuelled my desire to read more and get updated with relevant literature. My mind still continues to be troubled with various ideas, which are sometimes conflicting, when trying to devise management plans in complex atypical cases. Meanwhile, the theoretical exploration of all treatment options took the shape of this handbook with chapters written by some of the best minds in the business to deal with this crippling condition. It is for the first time that such an issue has been given the shape of a book with compilation of possibly all treatment options mentioned in the literature.

The initial nine chapters in this handbook focus on the problems of trigeminal neuralgia highlighting aetiopathogenesis and commonly available therapeutic options. One chapter is dedicated to the diagnostic and therapeutic radiological aspects in relation to the problem. Another nine chapters discuss about agents and procedures utilised for different peripheral nerve blocks and the complications thereof. The book includes chapters on commonly practiced percutaneous ablative procedures, such as radiofrequency thermocoagulation, glycerol rhizolysis, and balloon compression, which would further broaden the knowledge of pain physicians. There are descriptions on currently popular advanced management strategies like gamma knife radiosurgery and the use of botulinum neurotoxin. To complete all proposed treatment modalities for the readers, chapters on cryotherapy, neuromodulation, prolotherapy, and complementary medicinal practice are also included. Management of the problem in association with two special situations involving multiple sclerosis and pregnancy has also been enumerated. The last chapter discusses on outcome with different treatments offered and practical scope for the future.

I convey my heartfelt gratitude to all the authors and coauthors, who contributed immensely with lots of information on their respective topics. I am thankful to the director of AIIMS, Prof. Randeep Guleria, for permitting me to edit this book. I take this opportunity to thank my beloved teacher, Prof. Hari Hara Dash, for being the constant source of encouragement during my academic journey. I offer my sincere gratitude to Prof. Arvind Chaturvedi, Prof. R S Chouhan, faculty, senior residents, and technicians in the Department of Neuroanaesthesiology and Critical Care at AIIMS, New Delhi, for providing me with a conducive atmosphere to pursue pain management, apart from neuroanaesthesia and neurocritical care. My special thanks to my junior colleagues, Dr. Ritesh Lamsal and Dr. Siddharth Chavali, for helping me at different stages of preparation of this book. I am indebted to Dr. Naren Aggarwal, Dr. Eti Dinesh, and Ms. Beauty Christobel Gunasekaran of Springer Nature publications for guiding me to refine and develop the manuscripts into the current shape of a book. I acknowledge the silent influence of my elder brother, Dr. Lalit Mohan Rath, in my medical journey and the constant motivation of my father and parents-in-law for writing and editing scientific literature. Last but not the least, I thank my wife, Sarita, and son, Naman, for their unconditional support without which this project would have been too tough to complete.

I am reasonably sure this book will be an excellent companion not only to pain physicians, neurologists, neurosurgeons, and dental surgeons, who regularly attend to patients of trigeminal neuralgia in their clinics, but also to the patients and their relatives, who can get some idea on this troublesome illness and its treatment options. Despite our best efforts, there must be shortcomings in editing this book; I shall appreciate if the readers could send us their valuable feedbacks.

New Delhi, India Girija Prasad Rath

Contents

Part I Basics of Trigeminal Neuralgia

Introduction to Trigeminal Neuralgia 3
Ritesh Lamsal and Girija Prasad Rath

Anatomy of Trigeminal Nerve 11
Gyaninder Pal Singh

Etiopathogenesis of Trigeminal Neuralgia 23
Ashish Bindra

Clinical Presentation and Diagnosis of Trigeminal Neuralgia 31
Surya Kumar Dube

Differential Diagnosis of Trigeminal Neuralgia 37
Deepa Dash

Therapeutic Options for Trigeminal Neuralgia 45
Charu Mahajan

Radiology for Trigeminal Neuralgia 51
Pankaj Surange, Harshita Surange, and Gaurav Goyal

Pharmacotherapy of Trigeminal Neuralgia 63
Ayush Agarwal and Manjari Tripathi

Part II Peripheral Nerve Blocks for Trigeminal Neuralgia

Medications for Interventional Pain Management in Trigeminal Neuralgia 71
Siddharth Chavali

Supraorbital Nerve Block 79
Siddharth Chavali and Girija Prasad Rath

Supratrochlear Nerve Block 85
Siddharth Chavali and Girija Prasad Rath

Infraorbital Nerve Block 91
Siddharth Chavali and Girija Prasad Rath

Auriculotemporal and Zygomaticotemporal Nerve Block 97
Siddharth Chavali and Girija Prasad Rath

Mandibular Nerve Block for Trigeminal Neuralgia 103
Shiv Pratap Rana

Maxillary Nerve Block for Trigeminal Neuralgia 109
Shiv Pratap Rana

Mental Nerve Block 115
Siddharth Chavali and Girija Prasad Rath

Intra-Oral Nerve Blocks for Trigeminal Neuralgia 121
Rahul Yadav and Siddharth Chavali

Part III Surgical Treatment of Trigeminal Neuralgia

Glycerol Rhizolysis for Trigeminal Neuralgia 133
Hari Hara Dash

Radiofrequency Thermocoagulation for Trigeminal Neuralgia 141
Parmod Kumar Bithal

Percutaneous Microballoon Compression for Trigeminal Neuralgia. 151
Virender Kumar Mohan and Debesh Bhoi

Neurosurgical Treatment for Trigeminal Neuralgia 161
Sachin A. Borkar, Mohit Agrawal, and Sumit Sinha

Gamma Knife Radiosurgery for Trigeminal Neuralgia 169
Kanwaljeet Garg and Varidh Katiyar

Part IV Other Treatment Options for Trigeminal Neuralgia

Cryotherapy for Trigeminal Neuralgia 181
Ashish Bindra

Neuromodulation in Trigeminal Neuralgia 187
Ritesh Lamsal and Girija Prasad Rath

Botulinum Toxin for Trigeminal Neuralgia 195
Arunmozhimaran Elavarasi and Vinay Goyal

Neural Prolotherapy for Trigeminal Neuralgia 201
Ankur Khandelwal and Girija Prasad Rath

Complementary Medicine in Trigeminal Neuralgia 207
Rajeeb Kumar Mishra and Girija Prasad Rath

Part V Special Scenario with Trigeminal Neuralgia

Trigeminal Neuralgia in Multiple Sclerosis 217
Nitasha Mishra

Management of Trigeminal Neuralgia During Pregnancy 223
Bhanu Pratap Swain

Trigemino-Cardiac Reflex and Trigeminal Neuralgia. 231
Varun Jain and Gyaninder Pal Singh

Therapeutic Outcome and Future Scopes in the Management of Trigeminal Neuralgia 239
W. Umamaheshwara Rao and Muralidhar Joshi

About the Editor

Girija Prasad Rath is a Professor of Neuroanaesthesiology and Critical Care at Neurosciences Centre of All India Institute of Medical Sciences (AIIMS), New Delhi, India. He has received three years exclusive training in neuroanaesthesiology at AIIMS and is among the first batch of anaesthesiologists in India to hold a super-specialisation degree (DM-Neuroanaesthesiology). He is keenly interested in the education and clinical research activities related to neuroanaesthesia and neurocritical care. He has authored more than 200 scientific articles published in peer-reviewed journals of international repute. Dr. Rath is an editorial board member of the *Indian Journal of Anaesthesia* and has been working as the Executive Editor for the *Journal of Neuroanaesthesiology and Critical Care* (JNACC), since its inception. Dr. Rath is a Past Treasurer of Indian Society of Neuroanaesthesiology and Critical Care (ISNACC) and is an active member of international organisations like Society for Neuroscience in Anesthesiology and Critical Care (SNACC) and Asian Society for Neuroanesthesia and Critical Care (ASNACC). He is an invited speaker in the scientific meetings of various anaesthesia societies in India and abroad that includes EuroNeuro, World Congress of Anaesthesiologists (WCA), Neuroanaesthesia Symposium (NAS) of Malaysia, and ASNACC Singapore. Dr. Rath is a recipient of ICMR International Fellowship and is a Fellow of Indian College of Anaesthesiologists (FICA). His main areas of interest include awake craniotomy and neuroanaesthesia practices in children. Dr. Rath was involved in the first successful separation surgery of conjoined craniopagus twins in India and was felicitated for this achievement. He is also involved in the pain practice with special inclination towards the management of trigeminal neuralgia.

Part I

Basics of Trigeminal Neuralgia

Introduction to Trigeminal Neuralgia

Ritesh Lamsal and Girija Prasad Rath

Key Points

- Since pre-historic times, there have been several descriptions of human affliction from trigeminal neuralgia (TGN)
- Modern-day TGN therapy is the result of concerted effort invested in understanding the pathophysiology and treatment outcomes over several centuries
- Pharmacotherapy is the first line of management and microvascular decompression has excellent results in surgically amenable lesions
- Chemoneurolysis, balloon microcompression, radiofrequency lesioning. and stereotactic radiosurgery are other viable options with promising results

Synonyms

- Tic Douloureux
- Trifacial neuralgia
- Fothergill's disease or Fothergill neuralgia
- Prosopalgia or Prosoponeuralgia
- Suicide disease

R. Lamsal · G. P. Rath (✉)
Department of Neuroanaesthesiology and Critical Care Neurosciences Centre,
All India Institute of Medical Sciences, New Delhi, India

G. P. Rath (ed.), *Handbook of Trigeminal Neuralgia*,
https://doi.org/10.1007/978-981-13-2333-1_1

Overview

Trigeminal neuralgia (TGN) refers to recurrent lancinating pain that occurs in the distribution of one or more branches of the fifth cranial nerve. It is one of the commonest types of craniofacial pain disorders. The pain perception is typically unilateral, abrupt in onset, brief in duration, and usually starts after trivial stimuli. With progression of TGN, the interval between bouts of pain shorten. In advanced cases, patients may report of pain at most times of the day and pain relief with oral drugs may be very poor. The pain is most commonly felt in the distribution of maxillary (V_2) or mandibular (V_3) divisions of the trigeminal nerve [1]. Less common presentations include combinations of ophthalmic (V_1) and V_2, V_2 and V_3, or all three divisions [1]. Solitary involvement of V_1 division is very rare.

TGN has been classified by the International Classification of Headache Disorders-3 (2018) broadly into two types: (1) classical TGN, and (2) TGN due to other causes [1]. When the cause of neuralgia is a demonstrated or presumed loop of an aberrant blood vessel, it is known as "Classical TGN". Many other disease conditions can cause TGN, like acute herpes, post-herpetic neuralgia, post-traumatic neuralgia, multiple sclerosis and space-occupying lesions, such as cerebro-pontine angle tumor, arterio-venous malformation and meningioma.

Epidemiology

The overall incidence of TGN is about 40–50 cases per one million and estimated prevalence is approximately 100–200 per million population [2]. Incidence of TGN varies significantly with age, with less than 5 per million in people younger than 18 years, and some studies estimating as high as 800 per million in older age groups [3–5]. Patients in the age range of 35–65 years are most commonly affected [6]. For reasons that are not properly understood, TGN is nearly twice more common in females than males [7, 8]. Hereditary forms of TGN have been reported but are rare and constitute less than 4–5% of overall TGN [9]. However, patients with bilateral TGN have a higher hereditary predisposition than those with unilateral presentation [10]. Although there is no clear evidence, people with hypertension and migraine seem to be at an increased risk of developing TGN [7].

Early Historical Descriptions

The pain descriptions related to TGN have been extrapolated from written material available since pre-historic times. Early descriptions of this disorder can be inferred from the writings of renowned Roman and Greek physicians like Galen, Aretaeus and Cappadocia dating nearly two millennia back [11]. One of the earliest scientific notes of TGN was given by a German physician, Johannes Laurentius Bausch, in 1671 [12]. He suffered from TGN and later succumbed to the disease because of the inability to eat or drink properly. A few years later, John Locke, physician and philosopher, provided a detailed description of the disease including accounts of its treatment [13].

The pain associated with TGN can be so severe and disabling that it is sometimes also called the "**suicide disease**". Some old texts also refer to the disease as "**prosopalgia**", which is derived from two Greek words 'prosopon' (face) and 'algos' (pain). Severe bouts of TGN can trigger repetitive facial muscle spasms that mimic facial tics, giving rise to the name "***tic Douloureux***". This term was coined by Nicolas André in 1756 [13]. A more elaborate and scientific account of TGN was given by the distinguished English physician John Fothergill in the eighteenth century. He described it as "a painful affection of the face in sudden, sharp bouts, most commonly triggered by light touch or eating" [14]. TGN is also sometimes called the "***Fothergill's disease***". Several decades later, in the 1820s, Charles Bell localized this pain syndrome to the trigeminal nerve, after which the condition was known as "***Trigeminal Neuralgia***" [13].

Historical Evolution of Treatment

Early reports describe TGN as a dreaded disease with very poor response to treatment. There are suggestions of resting in a dark room, taking hot baths and even ingestion of wine to treat the disease in ancient texts [13].

Medical Management (Pharmacotherapy)

Medical drugs were the only widely acceptable mode of treatment up until the nineteenth century. Compounds historically used in treatment included quinine, mercury, camphor, opium, arsenic, ether and trichlorethylene. The response to treatment with these drugs was poor, short-lived, and sometimes accompanied by serious side-effects.

- 1940s: Bergouignan (1942) was the first to describe anti-epileptic medications for TGN treatment with sodium diphenylhydantoin [15].
- 1960s: The use of phenytoin was popular until the 1960s. In a landmark paper published in 1962, Blom proposed the use of carbamazepine for treating TGN [16]. Since then, several antiepileptics such as lamotrigine, clonazepam, valproate and gabapentin have been described.
- Currently, carbamazepine or oxcarbazepine are the first-line medical drugs used for TGN.

Percutaneous Chemoneurolysis

- 1800s: Early advocates of chemoneurolysis were Barthlow (1876), who described the benefits of injecting chloroform, and Neuber (1883), who promoted the use of osmic acid in the vicinity of the nerve trunks [13]. Neither technique gained widespread popularity.

- Early 1900s: In 1904, the first description of percutaneous technique using alcohol injections in the peripheral trigeminal nerve was given by Schloesser [17]. Several other caustic substances were injected into the gasserian ganglion over the ensuing years, such as phenol and other types of alcohol. A few years later, Pollock and Potter suggested the use of x-rays to confirm the position of injecting needle [13]. This concept of using imaging to minimize complications revolutionized the entire field of percutaneous procedures.
- 1980s: The efficacy of glycerol rhizotomy was established as a matter of serendipity in 1981. Häkanson was working to develop stereotactic gamma radiation, when he found that injection of glycerol, which was planned to be used only as a carrier medium, caused pain relief after injection into the trigeminal cistern, rather surprisingly [18].

Currently, the modern practitioners continue to use the same technique described by Häkanson with minor inter-personal modifications. Percutaneous procedures are popular because they are inexpensive, relatively safe in expert hands, and can be done as day-care cases.

Percutaneous Radiofrequency Lesioning

- Early 1900s: Radiofrequency (RF) lesioning of the TGN by electrocoagulation was described by Réthi in 1913 [19].
- 1930s: Stereotactic electrocoagulation of the Gasserian ganglion though the foramen ovale, using a specially designed head-frame, was first described by Kirschner in 1931 [20].
- 1970s: RF thermal lesioning of the trigeminal nerve was first performed by Sweet and Wepsic in 1974 [21]. The efficacy and safety of the procedure improved significantly because they also incorporated the idea of electrical stimulation for precise localization and temperature monitoring to prevent neuronal injury.
- 1990s: There was a sharp increase in the interest for RF lesioning in patients with TGN. Notable contributions for retrogasserian RF lesioning were made by Nugent [22] who used cordotomy-type electrodes, and Taha [23] by using thermistor-tipped electrodes.

Percutaneous Balloon Compression

- 1950s: Percutaneous balloon compression (PBC) originated from the pioneering works of Shelden and Pudenz in the 1950s [24]. There was high incidence of trauma to the vessels and surrounding brain tissue in some of these early attempts.
- 1980s: Mullan described a novel PBC technique of the fifth nerve ganglion using Fogarty balloon catheter in 1983 [25].

- 1990s and beyond: Several improvements in the original balloon compression technique were suggested by authors such as Brown during this period [26]. With improvement in the percutaneous needle sets and imaging modalities, PBC is currently considered safe and efficacious in majority of patients with drug-refractory TGN.

Stereotactic Gammaknife Radiosurgery

- 1970s: Lars Leksell first described the use of stereotactic-radiation targeting trigeminal ganglion. This minimally-invasive procedure consists of accurately delivering multiple rays of high-energy photons to destroy components of the trigeminal nerve root.
- 1990s and beyond: In 1993, a case series by Rand and colleagues, which showed significant improvement with stereotactic radiosurgery in majority of their patients with medically/surgically refractory TGN, without any notable complication, stimulated significant interest in this modality [27]. Currently, with improvement in high-precision imaging, retrogasserian gamma knife radiosurgery (GKRS) has become one of the mainstream methods of providing safe and efficacious treatment in patients with refractory lesions, or if the patient is unwilling/unfit for surgery. This modality holds a lot of promise in the days ahead.

Open Neurosurgery

Open surgical methods of treating TGN have existed even longer than the percutaneous methods. Early surgical descriptions date back to the 1750s, but without much success.

- 19th and early 20th centuries: The earliest surgical treatment of the trigeminal ganglion was given by Carcochan in 1858 [17]. With further refinement over the next several decades, the technique of selective sectioning of the affected fibers of the dorsal trigeminal root later became popular as the ***Spiller-Frazier technique***. This technique was introduced in the 1920s and widely practiced for over half a century [17].
- 1920s: Walter Dandy improved upon this technique and he was the first to note and comment on how impingement of arterial and venous vascular loops on the trigeminal nerve was present in many cases. This was a landmark observation in the understanding of the pathophysiology of TGN.
- 1950s: Palle Taarnhoj from Denmark and James Gardener from the USA were instrumental in building on the principles of Spiller, Frazier and Dandy and published large series of cases with excellent post-surgical outcomes.
- 1990s and beyond: The credit of further improvement of the surgical technique goes to Peter Jannetta with the advent of the operating microscope. He was able

to prove that anomalous vascular loops compressing the trigeminal nerve resulted in focal demyelination and alteration of neuronal physiology leading to the pain of TGN. After his publication of nearly 1200 cases in 1996, microvascular decompression (MVD) has been established as the surgical treatment of choice in classical TGN [28].

Conclusion

TGN is a dreadful disease, which can lead to incapacitating consequences. Descriptions of human suffering and attempts to understand and treat the disease have been ongoing for hundreds of years. Knowledge of the disease pathophysiology and better treatment modalities have surged in the last few decades. While the disease is still not understood in its entirety, use of modern therapeutic drugs, various percutaneous procedures, gamma knife surgery, and open neurosurgery have helped to successfully treat and alleviate the pain of TGN to a large extent.

References

1. Headache Classification Committee of the International Headache Society (IHS). The international classification of headache disorders, 3rd edition. Cephalalgia. 2018;38:1–211.
2. Manzoni GC, Torelli P. Epidemiology of typical and atypical craniofacial neuralgias. Neurol Sci. 2005;26(Suppl 2):s65–7.
3. Koopman JS, Dieleman JP, Huygen FJ, de Mos M, Martin CG, Sturkenboom MC. Incidence of facial pain in the general population. Pain. 2009;147:122–7.
4. Hall GC, Carroll D, Parry D, McQuay HJ. Epidemiology and treatment of neuropathic pain: the UK primary care perspective. Pain. 2006;122:156–62.
5. Hooge JP, Redekop WK. Trigeminal neuralgia in multiple sclerosis. Neurology. 1995;45:1294–6.
6. De Toledo IP, Conti Reus J, Fernandes M, Porporatti AL, Peres MA, Takaschima A, et al. Prevalence of trigeminal neuralgia: a systematic review. J Am Dent Assoc. 2016;147:570–6.e2.
7. Katusic S, Beard CM, Bergstralh E, Kurland LT. Incidence and clinical features of trigeminal neuralgia, Rochester, Minnesota, 1945-1984. Ann Neurol. 1990;27:89–95.
8. Maarbjerg S, Gozalov A, Olesen J, Bendtsen L. Trigeminal neuralgia – a prospective systematic study of clinical characteristics in 158 patients. Headache. 2014;54:1574–82.
9. Reddy GD, Viswanathan A. Trigeminal and glossopharyngeal neuralgia. Neurol Clin. 2014;32:539–52.
10. Pollack IF, Jannetta PJ, Bissonette DJ. Bilateral trigeminal neuralgia: a 14-year experience with microvascular decompression. J Neurosurg. 1988;68:559–65.
11. Pearce JM. Trigeminal neuralgia (Fothergill's disease) in the 17th and 18th centuries. J Neurol Neurosurg Psychiatry. 2003;74:1688.
12. Patel SK, Liu JK. Overview and history of trigeminal neuralgia. Neurosurg Clin N Am. 2016;3:265–76.
13. Cole CD, Liu JK, Apfelbaum RI. Historical perspectives on the diagnosis and treatment of trigeminal neuralgia. Neurosurg Focus. 2005;18:E4.
14. Fothergill J. Of a painful affection of the face. Medical observations and inquiries. 1773;5:129–42.
15. Bergouignan M. Cures heureuses de neurologies essentielles par le dephenyl hydantoinate de sounde. Rev Laryngol Otol Rhinol. 1942;63:34–41.

16. Blom S. Trigeminal neuralgia: its treatment with a new anticonvulsant drug (G-32883). Lancet. 1962;1:839–40.
17. Stookey B, Ransohoff J. Trigeminal neuralgia: its history and treatment. In: Thomas CP, editor. Principles of neurological surgery. Springfield, IL: Charles C. Thomas; 1959.
18. Lunsford LD, Bennett MH. Percutaneous retrogasserian glycerol rhizotomy for tic douloureux: part 1. Technique and results in 112 patients. Neurosurgery. 1984;14:424–30.
19. Wilkins R. Trigeminal neuralgia: historical overview, with emphasis on surgical treatment. In: Burchiel K, editor. Surgical management of pain. New York: Thieme; 2002. p. 288–301.
20. Kirschner M. Zur elektrochirurgie. Langenbecks Arch Klin Chir. 1931;167:761–8.
21. Sweet WH, Wepsic JG. Controlled thermocoagulation of trigeminal ganglion and rootlets for differential destruction of pain fibers. 1. Trigeminal neuralgia. J Neurosurg. 1974;40:143–56.
22. Nugent GR. Radiofrequency treatment of trigeminal neuralgia using a cordotomy-type electrode. A method. Neurosurg Clin N Am. 1997;8:41–52.
23. Taha JM, Tew JM Jr. Treatment of trigeminal neuralgia by percutaneous radiofrequency rhizotomy. Neurosurg Clin N Am. 1997;8:31–9.
24. Abdennebi B, Bouatta F, Chitti M, Bougatene B. Percutaneous balloon compression of the Gasserian ganglion in trigeminal neuralgia. Long-term results in 150 cases. Acta Neurochir. 1995;136:72–4.
25. Mullan S, Lichtor T. Percutaneous microcompression of the trigeminal ganglion for trigeminal neuralgia. J Neurosurg. 1983;59:1007–12.
26. Brown JA, Chittum CJ, Sabol D, Gouda JJ. Percutaneous balloon compression of the trigeminal nerve for treatment of trigeminal neuralgia. Neurosurg Focus. 1996;1:E10.
27. Rand RW, Jacques DB, Melbye RW, Copcutt BG, Levenick MN, Fisher MR. Leksell Gamma Knife treatment of tic douloureux. Stereotact Funct Neurosurg. 1993;61(Suppl 1):93–102.
28. Barker FG 2nd, Jannetta PJ, Bissonette DJ, Larkins MV, Jho HD. The long-term outcome of microvascular decompression for trigeminal neuralgia. N Engl J Med. 1996;334:1077–83.

Anatomy of Trigeminal Nerve

Gyaninder Pal Singh

Key Points

- Trigeminal nerve is the largest cranial nerve, and is a mixed nerve
- It is the principal sensory nerve for face and part of scalp, and gives motor supply to muscles of mastication
- Trigeminal ganglion is the largest sensory ganglion that lies within the Meckel's cave, and is the only sensory ganglion which is intracranial
- Various physiological reflexes (trigeminocardiac reflex, blink reflex, occulocardiac reflex, maxillomandibular reflex, diving reflex, and masseter reflex) are described in relation to trigeminal nerve
- Trigeminal neuralgia is a severe disabling condition where pain occurs in the distribution of one or more divisions of trigeminal nerve

Introduction

Trigeminal nerve is the fifth (V) cranial nerve and is also known as ***Trifacial nerve***. It is the largest of the twelve cranial nerves and has a broad territory of distribution. It is a mixed nerve with both motor and sensory fibers. The nerve originates from the brainstem (pons) and supplies various structures of the head and face. It is a paired nerve, and each nerve supply ipsilateral half of the head and face. Each trigeminal nerve has three main branches and so the name trigeminal (from Latin word "trigeminus" meaning three twins). The sensory modalities of the facial region are more complex and specialized than any other part of the body. There are zones of dense innervation in the

G. P. Singh (✉)
Department of Neuroanaesthesiology and Critical Care, All India Institute of Medical Sciences (AIIMS), New Delhi, India

G. P. Rath (ed.), *Handbook of Trigeminal Neuralgia*,
https://doi.org/10.1007/978-981-13-2333-1_2

territory of trigeminal nerve, and therefore have more number of neurons which explains the larger size of the trigeminal nerve compared to other nerves.

Functional Components

Trigeminal nerve has two functional components i.e. *special visceral or branchial efferent* (motor fibers) supplying the muscles derived from Ist branchial or pharyngeal arch and *general somatic afferent* (sensory fibers) carrying general sensations from head and face. The motor fibers originate from the motor nucleus of trigeminal whereas the sensory fibers terminate into the sensory nuclei of trigeminal in the brainstem. The components, function, central connections, location of cell bodies, and peripheral distribution of trigeminal nerve fibers are summarized in Table 1.

Trigeminal Nerve Nuclei

The sensory and motor nuclei of trigeminal nerve are located in the brainstem (Fig. 1). The sensory nucleus of trigeminal is a collection of three nuclei located in the midbrain, pons, medulla and upper two segments of cervical cord. These are

Table 1 Summary of the components, function, central connections, location of cell bodies, and peripheral distribution of trigeminal nerve fibers

Components	Function	Central connections	Location of cell bodies	Peripheral distribution
General Somatic Afferent (GSA)	General sensations (touch, pain, temperature)	Main Sensory Nucleus and Spinal Nucleus of V	Gasserian Ganglion	Sensory nerve endings to skin & mucous membrane of the head & face through ophthalmic, maxillary & mandibular nerves
	(Proprioception)	Mesencephalic Nucleus of V	Mesencephalic Nucleus of V	Sensory nerve endings in the muscles of mastication through mandibular nerve & in the extraocular muscles through ophthalmic nerve
Special Visceral Efferent (SVE)	Mastication	Motor Nucleus of V	Motor Nucleus of V	Motor nerve endings to temporalis, masseter, pterygoids, mylohyoid, tensor tympani, and tensor veli palatini through motor root of mandibular nerve

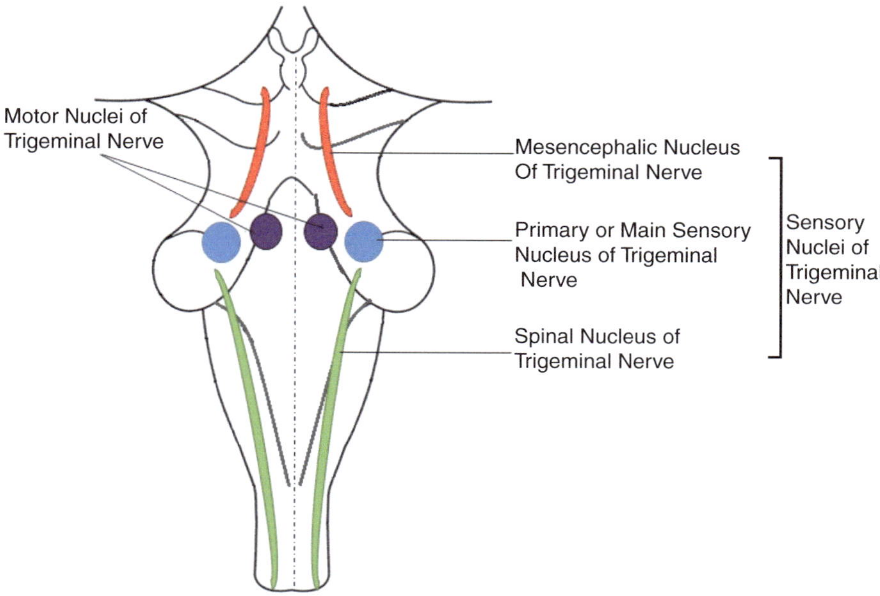

Fig. 1 Location of trigeminal nerve nuclei in the brainstem

the *mesencephalic nucleus* (in the midbrain), *principal or main sensory nucleus* (in the upper part of pons) and *spinal nucleus* (extending into the lower part of pons, medulla and upper two cervical segments of the spinal cord). The spinal nucleus is subdivided into three parts or sub-nuclei (i.e. the pars oralis, pars interpolaris and pars caudalis). The *motor nucleus* of the trigeminal nerve is located in the upper and dorsal part of pons, medial to the main sensory nucleus of trigeminal nerve.

The mesencephalic nucleus receives proprioceptive impulses from muscles of mastication, temporomandibular joint and probably from extraocular muscles. The main sensory nucleus receives touch sensation, and spinal nucleus receives pain and temperature sensation from the skin of head and face, mucous membrane of oral cavity, nasal cavity and paranasal sinuses, and meninges via the sensory root fibers. The motor nucleus supplies the derivatives of the first pharyngeal (mandibular) arch which includes muscles of mastication, mylohyoid, anterior belly of digastric, tensor veli palatini and tensor tympani via motor root fibers [1].

Trigeminal Roots and Nerve

The trigeminal nerve emerges from the ventrolateral surface of the pons at its junction with the middle cerebellar peduncle. It arises by a large lateral *sensory root* and a small medial *motor root* (Fig. 2). The point where the roots emerge from the brain

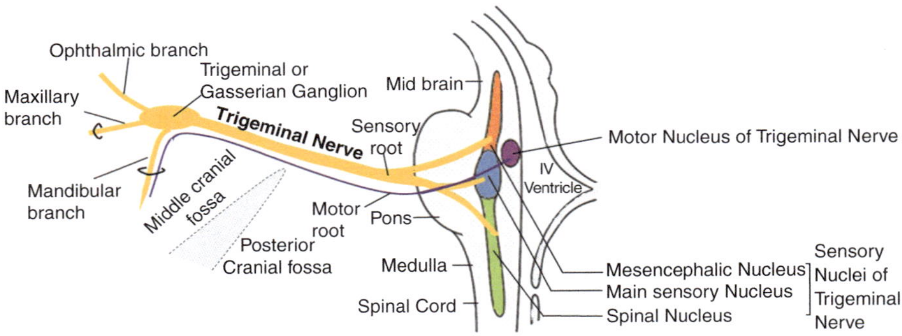

Fig. 2 Origin and course of trigeminal nerve

stem is known as ***root entry zone*** **(REZ)**. The fibers of the sensory root of the trigeminal nerve enter the pons and terminate into the sensory nuclei. The fibers of the motor nuclei form the motor root that emerge from the pons. The sensory and motor roots of trigeminal nerve are analogous to the dorsal (sensory) and ventral (motor) roots of the spinal nerves. The motor and sensory roots exist as separate bundles and together form the trigeminal nerve.

The trigeminal nerve passes forward, upwards and laterally from the posterior cranial fossa to reach the apex of the petrous part of the temporal bone in the middle cranial fossa. The nerve travels through the subarachnoid space from the pons into the Meckel's cave (described later) where the sensory root of the trigeminal nerve enlarges to form a crescentic structure known as the trigeminal ganglion (Fig. 2). The motor fibers lie below the sensory ganglion and do not entre the trigeminal ganglion. From the anterior aspect of the trigeminal ganglion arise the three peripheral branches of the trigeminal nerve viz: the ophthalmic, maxillary and mandibular branches (Fig. 2).

Trigeminal Ganglion

It is a sensory ganglion of the trigeminal nerve. It is the largest sensory ganglion of the body and the only sensory ganglion that lies inside the cranial cavity. It corresponds to the dorsal root ganglion (sensory) of a spinal nerve. Antonius Hirsh in 1965, first described this ganglion with the terminology **Gasserian ganglion** in honor of his teacher Johann Lorenz Gasser, an Austrian anatomist. The ganglion is an expansion of sensory root from the pons [2]. It is a crescent shaped structure with convex anterior margin, and so also known as **Semilunar Ganglion**. It lies in the floor of the middle cranial fossa in a small impression near the apex of petrous part of temporal bone [3, 4]. It invaginates a dural fold known as **Trigeminal or Meckel's Cave (Cavum Trigeminale)** that is formed by folding of meningeal layer of duramater around the ganglion [3–5] (Fig. 3).

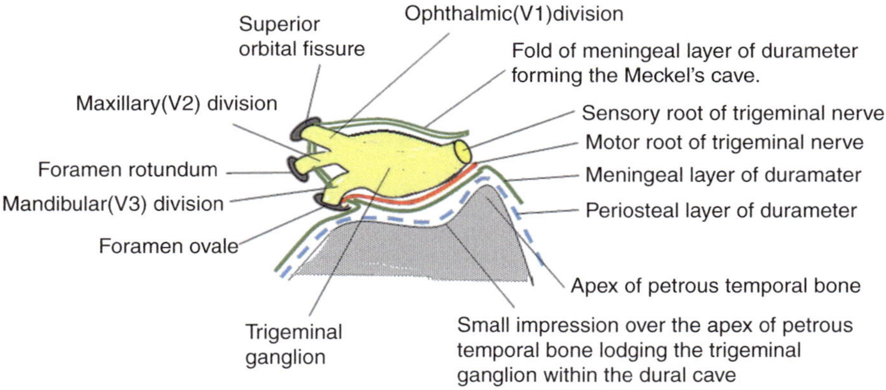

Fig. 3 Trigeminal ganglion in Meckel's cave

Branches of Trigeminal Nerve

There are three peripheral branches of the trigeminal nerve which arise from the anterior aspect (convex margin) of the trigeminal ganglion. These are the ophthalmic (V1), maxillary (V2) and mandibular (V3) nerves. These branches pierce the Meckel's cave and passes forward to exit the middle cranial fossa through small openings or foramen. Each of these three divisions further divides into multiple branches to supply various structures. The ophthalmic and maxillary divisions carry only sensory fibers whereas the mandibular division carries both sensory and motor fibers. Some of the peripheral branches also contain pre- or post-ganglionic parasympathetic and post ganglionic sympathetic fibers that supply the various glands of face, mouth, nose and eyes [6].

- **Ophthalmic Nerve** is a pure sensory nerve which originates from the anterolateral aspect of trigeminal ganglion. It is the smallest of the three divisions of trigeminal nerve. It lies in the lateral wall of the cavernous sinus and branches into the frontal, lacrimal and nasociliary nerves. All the three branches pass through the superior orbital fissure into the orbit. Within the cavernous sinus it also gives a meningeal branch and fine twigs to oculomotor, trochlear and abducens nerves that carry sensory fibers (proprioception) to extraocular muscles supplied by these nerves.
- **Maxillary Nerve** is a sensory branch which lies in the lateral wall of the cavernous sinus. It leaves the middle cranial fossa by passing through the foramen rotundum and enters the pterygopalatine fossa.
- **Mandibular Nerve** is the largest branch from the trigeminal ganglion. It immediately leaves the middle cranial fossa by passing through the foramen ovale and enters the temporal fossa. It is accompanied by the motor root of trigeminal nerve as it passes through the foramen oval and the two joins together in the

temporal fossa. Thus, the mandibular branch of the trigeminal nerve is a mixed nerve having both sensory and motor fibers.

Connections of Trigeminal Nerve Fibers

The afferent sensory neurons of the trigeminal nerve transmit sensory impulses. These are *pseudo-unipolar neurons* i.e. single process emerges from the cell body which divides into peripheral and central processes (Fig. 4). The cell bodies of these pseudo-unipolar neurons lie in the trigeminal ganglion and their processes pass into the trigeminal nerve and its branches. The peripheral processes of these neurons lie in the three peripheral branches of trigeminal nerve whereas the central processes pass in the sensory root of trigeminal nerve (Fig. 5). These are the *first order neurons* and they terminate in the main sensory nucleus and spinal nucleus of the trigeminal nerve. These neurons carry the touch, pain and temperature sensations. However, the pseudo-unipolar neurons which carry proprioceptive impulses from the muscles of mastication and extraocular muscles (*first order neuron*) have their cell body located in the mesencephalic nucleus of trigeminal nerve in the midbrain

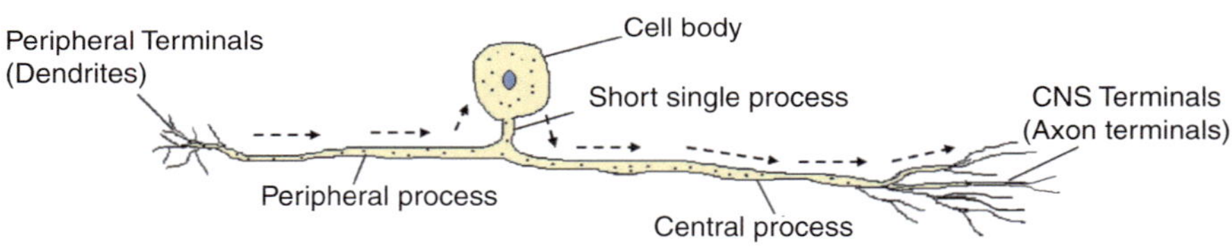

Fig. 4 Pseudo-unipolar neuron

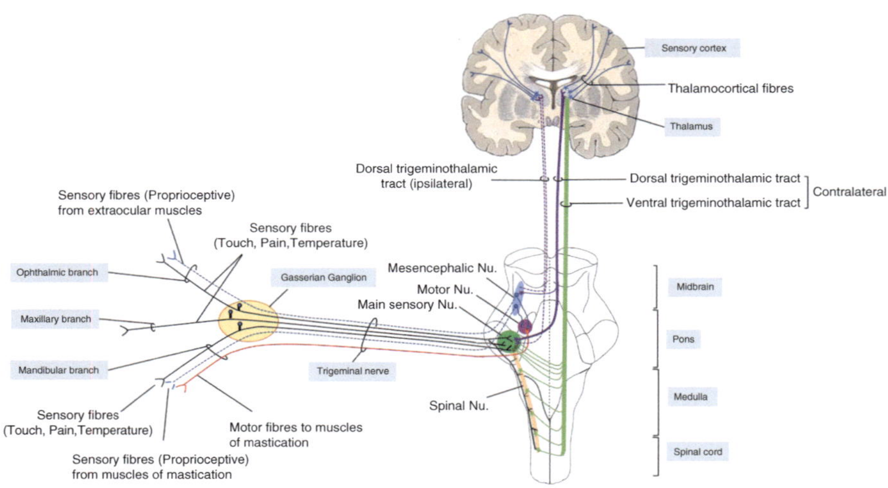

Fig. 5 Connections of trigeminal nerve fibers

(and not in the trigeminal ganglion) [6]. The peripheral process of these neurons travel from the muscles of mastication (muscle spindles) through the motor root of mandibular division, trigeminal ganglion and the trigeminal nerve to reach the cell bodies in mesencephalic nucleus (Fig. 5).

The first order neurons synapse with the *second order neurons* located in the sensory nucleus of trigeminal (mesencephalic, main sensory and spinal nucleus) in the brain stem. The axons of second order neurons cross to the opposite side and ascends in the *ventral and dorsal trigeminothalamic tracts* to relay in the *ventral postero-medial (VPM) nucleus* of the thalamus [6, 7]. The ventral (anterior) trigeminothalamic tract receives crossed fibers from contralateral main sensory and spinal nucleus of trigeminal and carry crude touch, pain and temperature sensations. The dorsal (posterior) trigeminothalamic tract mostly receives crossed fibers from the contralateral main sensory nucleus and few uncrossed fibers from ipsilateral main sensory nucleus and they carry fine touch and proprioceptive sensations. Both the anterior and posterior trigeminothalamic tracts projects to the VPM nucleus of thalamus. These fibers (second order neurons) synapse with neurons in the thalamus i.e. *third order neurons*. The axons of the third order neurons (thalamocortical fibers) project on to the sensory cerebral cortex posterior to the central sulcus [6, 7] (Fig. 5).

The first order neurons in the mesencephalic nucleus (proprioceptive fibers) have a short central process. These neurons synapse with the neurons in the motor nucleus of trigeminal nerve (forming reflex arch for jaw jerk or masseteric reflex) and with the second order neurons in the mesencephalic nucleus that carry proprioceptive impulse to the VPM nucleus of thalamus (via dorsal trigeminothalamic tracts) and then to the primary sensory cortex via thalamocortical fibers.

There are numerous intra- and inter-nuclear connections within the nuclei of trigeminal [8] and between the trigeminal nuclei and other brainstem nuclei [6]. The short internuncial neurons connect the sensory nucleus of trigeminal with other motor nuclei including oculomotor, trigeminal, facial, vestibular, glossopharyngeal, vagal, and hypoglossal. It also has connections with superior colliculus, and cerebellar cortex [9, 10]. In addition, there are neurons projecting from the cerebral cortex to the sensory and motor nucleus of trigeminal nerve in the brain stem (corticobulbar tracts) on each side. Most of these fibers are crossed (from contralateral cortex) and they have inhibitory function (inhibit sensory and motor nuclei of trigeminal nerve).

Areas Supplied by Trigeminal Nerve

The trigeminal nerve innervates various structures of head and face through its branches (Table 2). The areas supplied by the three primary divisions of trigeminal nerve is shown in Fig. 6. The Ophthalmic (V1) branch gives sensory supply to upper third of face including forehead, upper eyelid, conjunctiva, cornea, nose, nasal mucosa, frontal sinus, lacrimal gland and scalp up to vertex. It also forms the afferent limb of corneal reflex. The Maxillary (V2) branch supplies sensory fibers to middle third of the face including skin over temple, lower eyelid and conjunctiva, cheek, upper lip, nares, nasal mucosa, upper teeth and gums, maxillary sinus, mucous membrane of palate and pharynx, and dura mater of middle cranial fossa. Maxillary nerve also conveys secretomotor fibers to the lacrimal gland and the glands of palate, nose, maxillary sinus and oral cavity [11, 12]. The sensory fibers of Mandibular (V3) branch supplies the lower third of face including lower lip, chin, lower jaw except the small area over the angle of mandible, lower teeth and gums, part of auricle, temple, and part of meninges [11]. The motor fibers of V3 supply muscles of mastication (masseter, temporalis, medial and lateral pterygoid), mylohyoid, anterior belly of digastric, tensor veli palatini, and tensor tympani. Mandibular nerve forms both afferent and efferent limbs of jaw-jerk (masseter or masticatory) reflex.

Table 2 Areas innervated by the branches of trigeminal nerve

	Branches	Innervation
Trigeminal Ganglion	Meningeal branches	Duramater (middle cranial fossa, tentorium cerebelli)
Ophthalmic (V1) Nerve	Meningeal branches	Durameter (anterior cranial fossa tentorium cerebelli, falx cerebrii), superior sagittal sinus.
	Twigs to III, IV, VI CNs	Extraocular muscles (proprioceptive sensory fibers)
– Frontal nerve	Supraorbital neve	Upper eyelid, conjunctiva, forehead, Scalp
	Supratrochlear nerve	Upper eyelid, conjunctiva, forehead
– Nasociliary nerve	Anterior ethmoidal nerve	Mucous membranes of frontal, ethmoid and sphenoid sinuses, nasal cavity
	Posterior ethmoid nerve	Mucous membranes of sphenoid sinus
	Infratrochlear nerve	Bridge of nose, upper eyelid and conjunctiva
	Long ciliary nerves	Sensory innervation to eye (cornea, ciliary bodies, iris)
		Contains sympathetic fibers to dilator pupillae muscle
– Lacrimal nerve		Lacrimal gland, upper eyelid, conjunctiva
		Contains parasympathetic fibers to lacrimal gland
Maxillary (V2) Nerve	Middle meningeal branch	Duramater(middle cranial fossa) middle meningeal vessel
– Two branches to Pterygopalatine Ganglion (Pterygo-palatine nerves)	Nasopalatine nerve	Nasal cavity, palate Superior& middle turbinate, septum
	Pharyngeal nerve	Soft and hard palate, nasopharynx
	Greater Palatine nerve	Hard palate, palatal gingiva
	Lesser Palatine nerve	Nasopharynx, uvula, tonsil, soft palate

(continued)

Table 2 (continued)

	Branches	Innervation
– Zygomatic nerve	Zygomaticotemporal nerve	Skin over the temporal region, lacrimal gland (carry parasympathetic fibers from VII nerve to lacrimal gland)
	Zygomaticofacial nerve	Skin over the zygomatic bone, cheek
– Posterior superior alveolar nerve		Gingiva, maxilla, alveolar periosteum, maxillary teeth (molar, premolar), maxillary sinus, nasal floor
– Infraorbital nerve	Middle Superior Alveolar	Maxillary teeth (premolar), alveolar periosteum
	Anterior Superior Alveolar	Maxillary teeth (canine, incisors), alveolar periosteum
	Inferior Palpebral nerve	Lower eyelid, cheek
	External Nasal nerve	Nares
	Superior Labial nerve	Upper lip
Mandibular (V3) Nerve	Recurrent meningeal nerve	Duramater (middle cranial fossa)
	Medial pterygoid nerve	Medial pterygoid, tensor veli palatini, tensor tympani muscles
– Anterior division	Masseteric nerve	Masseter muscle, temporomandibular joint
	2 Deep temporal branches	Temporalis muscle
	Lateral pterygoid nerve	Lateral pterygoid muscle
	Buccinator nerve	Buccinator muscle
	Buccal nerve	Skin and mucous membrane of cheek and gingiva
– Posterior division	Auriculotemporal nerve	Skin of the auricle, meatus, and temporal region, tympanic membrane. Parasympathetic and sympathetic supply to the parotid gland after relay in the Otic ganglion
	Lingual nerve	Sensory to anterior tongue and gingiva. Taste sensations to the anterior 2/3 of tongue and parasympathetic fibers to facial nerve (communicates with VII CN)
	Inferior alveolar nerve	
	– Mylohyoid branch	Mylohyoid, anterior belly of digastric muscle
	– Dental branches	Lower molars, premolars, canine, gingiva
	– Incisive branch	Lower incisors, gingiva
	– Mental branch	Skin of chin, lower lip, gingiva

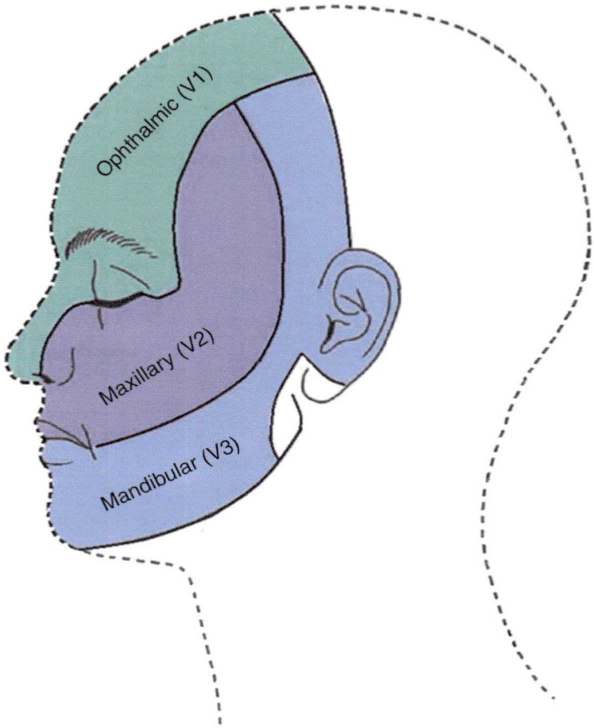

Fig. 6 Sensory distribution of three primary divisions of the trigeminal nerve

Clinical Significance

The trigeminal nerve is associated with various clinical conditions of head and face regions. ***Trigeminal Neuralgia (TGN)* or *Tic Douloureux*** presents with severe pain in the area of distribution of one or more divisions of the trigeminal nerve. It more frequently involves maxillary and mandibular divisions of the trigeminal nerve then the ophthalmic division. Compression of the nerve by vascular loops may lead to TGN [13–15]. There is a higher prevalence of pain on the right side which may probably be explained by the fact that the foramen rotundum and ovale are significantly narrower on right side as compared to left which may lead to easy compression on the nerves on right side [16]. Other painful condition in the distribution of trigeminal nerve may be trigeminal *postherpetic neuralgia* presenting with cutaneous allodynia and hyperalgesia.

Sensory deficit (hypoesthesia) in the territory of supratrochlear and supraorbital nerve may occur due to injury to these nerves or following surgery in prone position due to pressure on forehead and compression of these nerves by improperly positioned head rest. Injury to infraorbital branch of maxillary nerve may cause ***Numb Cheek Syndrome*** [17] and to mental nerve may cause ***Numb Chin***

Syndrome [18, 19]. Lesion of the motor root of trigeminal nerve may lead to ***Hemimasticatory Spasm*** characterized by recurrent spasm of masseters and temporalis muscle on one side [20].

In ***Lateral medullary syndrome*** (*Wallenberg Syndrome* or *Posterior Inferior Cerebellar Artery (PICA) Syndrome),* there occurs loss of pain and temperature sensation on ipsilateral side of the face and on contralateral side of the body. The ascending spinothalamic tract which carries pain and temperature sensation from contralateral side of body lies adjacent to descending spinal tract of trigeminal nerve carrying pain and temperature sensation from ipsilateral face, and hence, the effect. The PICA supplies the lower cerebellum, lateral medulla, and choroid plexus of the fourth ventricle. Infarction due to interrupted blood supply to lateral medulla after occlusion of PICA or vertebral artery may cause this syndrome [21, 22].

Trigeminal nerve is associated with several neurophysiological reflexes such as ***Trigeminal blink reflex, Trigeminocardiac reflex, Occulocardiac reflex, Maxillomandibular reflex, Diving reflex, Sucking reflex, Masseter reflex (Jaw jerk)*** each of which has its clinical significance. ***Marcus Gunn phenomenon*** (**Marcus-Gunn jaw-winking** or **trigemino-oculomotor synkineses**) and ***Inverse Marcus Gunn phenomenon*** (or **Marin-Amat syndrome**) are some of the other conditions associated with this nerve.

References

1. Romanes GJ. The peripheral nervous system: trigeminal nerve. In: Romanes GJ, editor. Cunningham's textbook of anatomy. 12th ed. Oxford, UK: Oxford University Press; 1981. p. 748–56.
2. Jannetta PJ. Gross (mesoscopic) description of the human trigeminal ganglion. J Neurosurg. 1967;26:109–11.
3. Joo W, Yoshioka F, Funaki T, Mizokami K, Rhoton AL Jr. Microsurgical anatomy of the trigeminal nerve. Clin Anat. 2014;27:61–88.
4. Soeira G, Abd el-Bary TH, Dujovny M, Slavin KV, Ausman JI. Microsurgical anatomy of the trigeminal nerve. Neurol Res. 1994;16:273–83.
5. Kapila A, Chakeres DW, Blanco E. The Meckel cave: computed tomographic study. Part I: normal anatomy; Part II: pathology. Radiology. 1984;152:425–33.
6. Liu GT. The Trigeminal nerve and its central connections. In: Miller NR, Newman NJ, Biousse V, Kerrison JB, editors. Walsh and Hoyt's clinical neuro-ophthalmology. 6th ed. Philadelphia, PA: Lippincott Williams & Wilkins; 2005. p. 1233–68.
7. Smith RD. Axonal projections and connections of the principal sensory trigeminal nucleus in the monkey. J Comp Neurol. 1975;163:347–76.
8. Ikeda M, Tanami T, Matsushita M. Ascending and descending internuclear connections of the trigeminal sensory nuclei in the cat. A study with the retrograde and anterograde horseradish peroxidase technique. Neuroscience. 1984;12:1243–60.
9. Silverman JD, Kruger L. Projections of the rat trigeminal sensory nuclear complex demonstrated by multiple fluorescent dye retrograde transport. Brain Res. 1985;361:383–8.
10. Steindler DA. Trigeminocerebellar, trigeminotectal, and trigeminothalamic projections: a double retrograde axonal tracing study in the mouse. J Comp Neurol. 1985;237:155–75.
11. Rodella LF, Buffoli B, Labanca M, Rezzani R. A review of the mandibular and maxillary nerve supplies and their clinical relevance. Arch Oral Biol. 2012;57:323–34.
12. Tomaszewska IM, Zwinczewska H, Gładysz T, Walocha JA. Anatomy and clinical significance of the maxillary nerve: a literature review. Folia Morphol. 2015;74:150–6.

13. Lang E, Naraghi R, Tanrikulu L, Hastreiter P, Fahlbusch R, Neundorfer B, Troscher-Weber R. Neurovascular relationship at the trigeminal root entry zone in persistent idiopathic facial pain: findings from MRI 3-D visualization. J Neurol Neurosurg Psychiatry. 2005;76:1506–9.
14. Bakshi R, Lerner A, Fritz JV, Sambuchi GD. Vacular compression in trigeminal neuralgia shown by magnetic resonance imaging and magnetic resonance angiography image registration. Arch Neurol. 2001;58:1290–1.
15. Dzierżanowski J, Słoniewski P. Trigeminal neuralgia caused by aneurysm of the posterior cerebral artery: a case description and the analysis of anatomical variety of vascular complex in the rood entry zone of trigeminal nerve. Folia Morphol. 2014;73:224–8.
16. Neto HS, Camilli JA, Marques MJ. Trigeminal neuralgia is caused by maxillary and mandibular nerve entrapment: greater incidence of right-sided facial symptoms is due to the foramen rotundum and foramen ovale being narrower on the right side of the cranium. Med Hypotheses. 2005;65:1179–82.
17. Campbell WW Jr. The numb cheek syndrome: a sign of infraorbital neuropathy. Neurology. 1986;36:421–3.
18. Bruyn RPM, Boogerd W. The numb chin. Clin Neurol Neurosurg. 1991;93:187–93.
19. Burt RK, Sharfman WH, Karp BI, Wilson WH. Mental neuropathy (numb chin syndrome). A harbinger of tumor progression or relapse. Cancer. 1992;70:877–81.
20. Cruccu G, Inghilleri M, Berardelli A, Pauletti G, Casali C, Coratti P, Frisardi G, Thompson PD, Manfredi M. Pathophysiology of hemimasticatory spasm. J Neurol Neurosurg Psychiatry. 1994;57:43–50.
21. Sacco RL, Freddo L, Bello JA, Odel JG, Onesti ST, Mohr JP. Wallenberg's lateral medullary syndrome: clinical-magnetic resonance imaging correlations. Arch Neurol. 1993;50:609–14.
22. Kim JS. Pure lateral medullary infarction: clinical-radiological correlation of 130 acute, consecutive patients. Brain. 2003;126:1864–72.

Etiopathogenesis of Trigeminal Neuralgia

Ashish Bindra

Key Points

- Pain in Trigeminal neuralgia (TGN) is attributed to dysfunctional hyperactivity of trigeminal nerve
- The commonest cause is a vascular loop compressing the nerve root entry zone (REZ); other causes of compression may include tumors, vascular malformations, and cysts
- TGN is also a common manifestation of multiple sclerosis
- Long-standing compression at REZ may cause focal demyelination, cross connection between the nerves fibers, and generation of abnormal electrical impulses

Introduction

Trigeminal neuralgia (TGN) is characterized by sudden, usually unilateral, recurrent lancinating pain arising from one or more divisions of the trigeminal nerve. It is a well-known medical condition for quite some time, but its etiopathogenesis is yet to be fully understood. The diagnosis is based on subjective pain perception rather than laboratory findings. The characteristic signs and symptoms, and response to distinctive set of therapeutic modalities helps not only in disease identification but also unveils the underlying pathogenetic mechanism. TGN is significantly more common with advancing age, and nearly twice as common in women than men [1]. Understanding the etiopathogenesis of the condition is important for proper

A. Bindra (✉)
Department of Neuroanaesthesiology and Critical Care, All India Institute of Medical Sciences (AIIMS), New Delhi, India

G. P. Rath (ed.), *Handbook of Trigeminal Neuralgia*,
https://doi.org/10.1007/978-981-13-2333-1_3

management and elimination of contributing factors. Unfortunately, many of the patients may not have an identifiable cause and disease remains mainly **idiopathic**. This chapter will summarise the etiopathogenesis of TGN.

Etiology

Many causative factors have been proposed, the main etiological factors contributing to development of TGN as supported by the literature are discussed below (Table 1).

1. **Direct Trauma or Compression of the Trigeminal Nerve**: The most commonly accepted theory is compression of trigeminal nerve root adjacent to pons at the dorsal root entry zone (REZ) as the cause of neuralgic pain [2, 3]. Vascular loop, arteriovenous malformation (AVM), aneurysm, tumors such as posterior fossa meningiomas, vestibular schwannoma, epidermoid, or tuberculoma, distortion of contents of posterior fossa by arachnoid cyst, or cranio-vertebral junction anomaly (CVJ) anomaly result in direct compression or compression of nerve against skull base. Tumors contribute to 2% of the cases of TGN [4]. The tumor which stretches the trigeminal nerve REZ results in neuralgic pain whereas the tumor involving the peripheral branches of the trigeminal ganglion result in constant pain instead of neuralgic pain.

   According to **Neurovascular Compression (NVC) Theory**, vascular loop is the cause of neuralgia in 80–90% of the cases. The most common vessel involved is superior cerebellar artery (SCA) in 85% of cases followed by anterior inferior cerebellar artery (AICA), posterior inferior cerebellar artery (PICA), and vertebral artery (VA) [5, 6]. In some cases, venous loop can be the additional or sole cause of compression [4, 5]. Haines and colleagues studied the vascular relationships of trigeminal REZ in 20 cadavers of individuals without any facial pain and 20 patients being operated for TGN. A total of 40 nerves were studied in each group. Nerve contact was common in cadavers but only few showed evidence of compression or distortion of nerve. Whereas majority of patients with TGN showed compression by adjacent arteries. Venous compression was seen in four of the cadaveric nerves and in eight nerves from patients with TGN. These data support the hypothesis that arterial compression of trigeminal nerve is associated

Table 1 Etiology of trigeminal neuralgia

Compressive Etiology	Systemic Diseases	Others
• **Vascular loop** • Tumors • Arteriovenous malformations • CVJ anomaly • Following surgical interventions? • Narrowing of osseous canals? • Rough bony margins?	• **Multiple sclerosis** • Diabetes Mellitus? • Vascular disease? • Hypertension?	• **Idiopathic** • Polyetiogenic? • Allergic?

with TGN [7]. Due to laminar arrangement of nerve fibres inside the trigeminal nerve the medial impingement by the vessel leads to V2 symptoms, lateral or caudal compression causes V3 symptoms, and rarely cranial compression, results in V1 symptoms [8]. Severe NVC is much more prevalent in men than in women [9]. Since vascular loop is the commonest cause of TGN, therefore, all newly diagnosed cases should undergo a magnetic resonance imaging (MRI) to rule out vascular impingement around the nerve [2, 10]. Nevertheless, vascular loop does not explain occurrence of symptoms in all the cases. Demonstrable vascular loops have also proven to be asymptomatic many times.

2. **Systemic Disease-Related Causes**
   Multiple Sclerosis (MS) is commonly associated with sensory disturbance (painless paraesthesia) as well as facial pain which may or may not be due to TGN. The trigeminal nerve may be affected secondary to MS [11]. The association between MS and TGN is not as common as it is thought of. TGN is reported to occur only in 0.9–4.5% of patients with MS. Conversely, 1.7–15% of patients diagnosed with TGN had associated MS [12]. In a few cases, TGN is the first symptom of MS. These patients are young and have bilateral presentation of TGN [13]. MR studies have shown demylelinating lesion at pontine trigeminal REZ. A high incidence of trigeminal involvement is seen in patients with MS, but lesions other than REZ are not associated with TGN and may remain clinically silent [14]. There is insufficient evidence to support MS as a primary cause of TGN. In an interesting case series of seven patients with MS, two patients had bilateral TGN, in patients with unilateral disease three patients had a vascular loop pressing the REZ, one had an epidermoid tumor whereas only one patient had a demyelinating lesion [15]. High-resolution MRI at 3T may yield a greater prevalence of detectable trigeminal abnormality in MS patients; however MRI findings might not correspond to trigeminal symptoms [16]. To summarize, there is still insufficient evidence to suggest MS as primary cause of TGN. TGN in patients with MS can be due to the demyelinating lesion or vascular compression at REZ [17].

   Other systemic ailments like **vascular disease, rheumatism, diabetes mellitus** etc. may play an additional role in development of neuralgia. According to few studies, there is a increased risk of developing TGN after **hypertension** [18, 19]. TGN is commonly accompanied by **atherosclerosis** and **arterial hypertonia**. The functional and morphological changes due to systemic disease leading to alteration in vascular supply of either peripheral branches or central origin of trigeminal nerve may contribute to neuralgia. However, a study done in cadavers of patients with vascular disease prove that there is no direct association between the neuralgia and vascular disease [20].
3. **Miscellaneous Causes**: Some authors report onset of TGN **following surgical interventions** unrelated to the trigeminal nerve, suggesting individual susceptibility, postoperative pressure and changes in cerebrospinal fluid flow leading to contact of trigeminal nerve with vascular structure as a cause of neuralgic pain [21]. Though there is no reasonable consideration that allergy could be responsible for TGN, an **allergic hypothesis** has ben proposed due to remissions, exacerbations,

and presence of provocative and relieving factors. The hypothesis remains largely unsupported by literature. Response to dental and otorhinolaryngology inflammation was said to be responsible for allergic reaction. High level of serum histamine, degranulating mast cells and conglomerates of immune complexes in peripheral part of trigeminal nerve were observed by Wang and collegues. During remission, mast cells were absent in the resected nerve trunks [22, 23]. Narrowing of osseous canals at exit of corresponding nerve branch is another enumerated cause of TGN [24]. Other theories include endogenous and exogenous intoxication, temporomandibular joint pathology and high position of petrous pyramid apex of temporal bone. Aggressive bony edges and acute bony angle of petrous ridge may also contribute to neuralgia specially in cases where there is no other demonstrable pathology [25]. A small cerebellopontine angle cistern area and shorter trigeminal nerve cisternal length may also play a role in the pathogenesis of TGN [26].

Pathophysiology

None of the existing theories explain all the characteristics of the disease. Neurovascular compression (NVC) resulting in morphological and structural changes is widely believed to cause neuralgic pain. Trigeminal nerve is the prime generator of pain. The peripheral pathogenetic mechanism produces progressive dystrophy and dysfunction of the nerve. Dorsal REZ, also known as **Redlich–Obersteiner's Zone** is the boundary between central and peripheral nervous systems. It corresponds to the junction of myelin of schwann cells with that of the glial cells (myelin of oligodendrocytes), and can be visually identified with a length of approximately 1.0–2.5 mm [2, 27]. REZ is often the place for NVC. The central branches of unipolar ganglion cells enter pons and arrive at brainstem and spinal nuclei through this transition zone. Long-standing compression at REZ results in alteration in neural function, membrane instability and demyelination. The interconnection between demyelinated neurons results in spontaneous activity and ectopic impulse generation. Development of TGN is a slow response to neural compression by a vascular loop, tumor or demyelinating plaque at REZ.

Initially, it was thought to be a functional disease without anatomical changes but later Kerr and colleagues observed morphological changes like interstitial neuritis, neural fibre demyelination and perineural and endoneural sclerosis in REZ samples of patients who underwent rhizotomy [28]. Nerve deviation, distortion, groove formation, and atrophy can be seen with high resolution imaging. Atrophic changes in trigeminal nerve are shown to correlate with severity of compression. Such changes also correlate with clinical outcomes and may help to predict long-term prognosis after vascular decompression. The demyelinated axons are in direct apposition, with few intervening glial processes. The proposed ***'short connection theory'*** suggests demyelination and cross talk as primary pathology causing spontaneous neuralgic pain [29]. Thin myelinated A-delta nociceptive fibres are predominantly susceptible to pressure changes. Pressure on these fibres result in ectopic generation of spontaneous nerve impulse and abnormal non-synaptic transmission to adjacent fibers.

Pulsatile mechanical compressions by the vessel may itself result in aberrant impulses within the demyelinated axons. The fibres transmitting light touch and pain are in closest proximity with REZ and causes paroxysmal pain provoked by cutaneous stimuli [2, 7]. AEDs help dampen abnormal electrical discharges and thus ameliorate the symptoms.

Although focal demyelination has been observed in the area of vascular contact, it does not occur in all individuals with vascular contact. Hence, few clinicians believe that there must be some individual susceptibility which predisposes to the development of focal demyelination at REZ and that mere vascular contact need not result in TGN.

The demyelinating lesions of MS at proximal part of trigeminal nerve results in neuralgic pain, wheras lesions in other part of the nerve or ganglion might not lead to such symptoms. Active demyelination changes including lipid laden macrophages are seen in histopathology samples of proximal nerve fibres.

According to ***Ignition Hypothesis*** [30], TGN results from specific abnormalities of afferent neurons in the trigeminal root or ganglion. Injury results in hyperexcitation of axons and axotomized somata. The synchronous firing of these hyperexcitable afferents, give rise to pain paroxysms. This hypothesis has been supported by study of abnormal electrical behaviour in injured sensory neurons and the findings from histopathologic observations obtained from patients with TGN, who underwent microvascular decompression surgery [12, 30].

Few researchers proposed **Central Pathogenetic Mechanism** as the cause of TGN. Central structures like thalamus, trigeminal nerve nuclei or cerebral cortical injury act as sites of origin of neuralgic pain [29]. According to this theory, TGN is a multineuronal reflex involving trigeminal and facial nerves, reticular formation, diencephalic nucleus and cerebral cortex. Afferent physiologic stimulation of trigeminal nerve receptors induces paroxysmal excitation focus on central structures and generates efferent impulses to peripheries. However, the structures generating long prethreshold impulses from peripheries and central structures of the trigeminal nerve responding by paroxysmal type discharge are not well defined. According to pathologic specimens studied from patients with TGN, the acute period of neuralgia induces dystrophy in peripheral neural fibres whereas in the subacute phase signs of regeneration are seen and number of fibres with dystrophy decrease. Gradually connective tissue replaces destroyed neural fibres and condition worsens with each exacerbation of disease. The nerve is involved in a retrograde manner, and gradually all peripheral branches are involved [31].

Conclusion

Trigeminal neuralgia is a debilitating condition. A patient of trigeminal neuralgia should be evaluated for all possible etiological factors. Vascular loop is the commenst cause of neuralgic patient. Other structural lesions like tumor, cysts or bony abnormality compressing the nerve root should also be recognized. Patients with MS may present with TGN. Thorough evaluation of such patients may help diagnose the systemic pathology, however, some patients might not have any identifiable etiology. Since the disease is diagnosed on the based on subjective pain perception rather than laboratory findings, a thorough history taking and clinical examination is corner stone of management. MRI should be done to rule out compressive pathology in all suspected cases.

References

1. Rothman KJ, Monson RR. Epidemiology of trigeminal neuralgia. J Chronic Dis. 1973;26:2–12.
2. Jannetta PJ. Vascular compression is the cause of TN. APS J. 1993;2:217–27.
3. Prasad S, Galetta S. Trigeminal neuralgia: historical notes and current concepts. Neurologist. 2009;15:87–94.
4. Nurmiko TJ, Eldridge PR. Trigeminal neuralgia: pathophysiology, diagnosis and current treatment. Br J Anaesth. 2001;87:117–32.
5. Yoshino N, Akimoto H, Yamada I, Nagaoka T, Tetsumura A, Kurabayashi T, Honda E, Nakamura S, Sasaki T. Trigeminal neuralgia: evaluation of neuralgic manifestation and site of neurovascular compression with 3D CISS MR imaging and MR angiography. Radiology. 2003;228:539–45.
6. de Lange EE, Vielvoye GJ, Voormolen JH. Arterial compression of the fifth cranial nerve causing trigeminal neuralgia: angiographic findings. Radiology. 1986;158:721–7.
7. Haines SJ, Jannetta PJ, Zorub DS. Microvascular relations of the trigeminal nerve. An anatomical study with clinical correlation. J Neurosurg. 1980;52:381–6.
8. Loesar JD. Trigeminal neuralgia. In: Bonica J, Ballantyne J, Fishman S, Rathmell J, editors. Bonica's management of pain. 3rd ed. Philadelphia: Lippincott, Williams & Wilkins; 2008.
9. Maarbjerg S, Wolfram F, Gozalov A, Olesen J, Bendtsen L. Association between neurovascular contact and clinical characteristics in classical trigeminal neuralgia: a prospective clinical study using 3.0 Tesla MRI. Cephalalgia. 2015;35:1077–84.
10. Love S, Coakham HB. Trigeminal neuralgia: pathology and pathogenesis. Brain. 2001;124:2347–60.
11. Burkholder DB, Koehler PJ, Boes CJ. Trigeminal neuralgia and multiple sclerosis: a historical perspective. Can J Neurol Sci. 2017;44:589–93.
12. Sabalys G, Juodzbalys G, Wang HL. Aetiology and pathogenesis of trigeminal neuralgia: a comprehensive review. J Oral Maxillofac Res. 2013;3:e2.
13. da Silva CJ, da Rocha AJ, Mendes MF, Maia AC Jr, Braga FT, Tilbery CP. Trigeminal involvement in multiple sclerosis: magnetic resonance imaging findings with clinical correlation in a series of patients. Mult Scler. 2005;11:282–5.
14. Meaney JF, Watt JW, Eldridge PR, Whitehouse GH, Wells JC, Miles JB. Association between trigeminal neuralgia and multiple sclerosis: role of magnetic resonance imaging. J Neurol Neurosurg Psychiatry. 1995;59:253–9.
15. Mills RJ, Young CA, Smith ET. Central trigeminal involvement in multiple sclerosis using high-resolution MRI at 3T. Br J Radiol. 2010;83:493–8.
16. Gass A, Kitchen N, MacManus DG, Moseley IF, Hennerici MG, Miller DH. Trigeminal neuralgia in patients with multiple sclerosis: lesion localization with magnetic resonance imaging. Neurology. 1997;49:1142–4.
17. Pan SL, Yen MF, Chiu YH, Chen LS, Chen HH. Increased risk of trigeminal neuralgia after hypertension: a population-based study. Neurology. 2011;77:1605–10.
18. Sandell T, Holmen J, Eide PK. Hypertension in patients with cranial nerve vascular compression syndromes and comparison with a population-based cohort. J Neurosurg. 2013;119:1302–8.
19. Smoliar E, Smoliar A, Sorkin L, Belkin V. Microcirculatory bed of the human trigeminal nerve. Anat Rec. 1998;250:245–9.
20. Duransoy YK, Mete M, Akcay E, Selcuki M. Differences in individual susceptibility affect the development of trigeminal neuralgia. Neural Regen Res. 2013;8:1337–42.

21. Wang X, Liang H, Zhou C, Xu M, Xu L. Sensitization induces hypersensitivity in trigeminal nerve. Clin Exp Allergy. 2012;42:1638–42.
22. Cui W, Yu X, Zhang H. The serotonin transporter gene polymorphism is associated with the susceptibility and the pain severity in idiopathic trigeminal neuralgia patients. J Headache Pain. 2014;15:42.
23. Sicard A. [Bernard Pierson 1925–1978]. Arch Anat Cytol Pathol. 1978;26:79–80. [Medline: 371549].
24. Brinzeu A, Dumot C, Sindou M. Role of the petrous ridge and angulation of the trigeminal nerve in the pathogenesis of trigeminal neuralgia, with implications for microvascular decompression. Acta Neurochir. 2018;160(5):971–6. https://doi.org/10.1007/s00701-018-3468-1.
25. Alfieri A, Fleischhammer J, Strauss C, Peschke E. The central myelin-peripheral myelin transitional zone of the nervus intermedius and its implications for microsurgery in the cerebellopontine angle. Clin Anat. 2012;25:882–8.
26. Parise M, Acioly MA, Ribeiro CT, Vincent M, Gasparetto EL. The role of the cerebellopontine angle cistern area and trigeminal nerve length in the pathogenesis of trigeminal neuralgia: a prospective case-control study. Acta Neurochir. 2013;155:863–8.
27. Kerr FW. Pathology of trigeminal neuralgia: light and electron microscopic observations. J Neurosurg. 1967;26(Suppl):151–6.
28. Dott NM. Facial pain: review of aetiological factors. Proc R Soc Med. 1951;44:1034.
29. Devor M, Amir R, Rappaport ZH. Pathophysiology of trigeminal neuralgia: the ignition hypothesis. Clin J Pain. 2002;18:4–13.
30. Rappaport ZH, Devor M. Trigeminal neuralgia: the role of self-sustaining discharge in the trigeminal ganglion. Pain. 1994;56:127–38.
31. Hanes WJ. Clinical research on the etiology and treatment of tic douloureux on an allergic basis. Report of 183 cases. Oral Surg Oral Med Oral Pathol. 1967;23:728–36.

Clinical Presentation and Diagnosis of Trigeminal Neuralgia

Surya Kumar Dube

Key Points

- Trigeminal neuralgia (TGN) is characterized by paroxysms of sudden, severe, electric current-like pain in the distribution of the trigeminal nerve
- Pain may arise spontaneously, or following a trigger
- TGN commonly involves the maxillary or mandibular divisions of the trigeminal nerve
- Pain is usually unilateral; bilateral presentation is rare, and right side is more commonly affected than the left

Introduction

Trigeminal neuralgia (TGN) is defined by the International Association for the Study of Pain (IASP) as "unilateral painful orofacial condition characterised by brief duration of electric shock-like sensation with an abrupt onset and termination, and limited to one or more sensory divisions of the trigeminal nerve". The pain may arise spontaneously, or may be triggered by innocuous mechanical stimuli and movement [1]. The International Headache Society (IHS) has described TGN more elaborately, and has suggested clinical criteria for the diagnosis of TGN. According to these suggestions, TGN is a medical condition characterized by paroxysmal attacks of sudden-onset, severe, shock-like, recurrent pain, along the distribution of one or more branches of the trigeminal nerve [2, 3].

S. K. Dube (✉)
Department of Neuroanaesthesiology and Critical Care, All India Institute of Medical Sciences (AIIMS), New Delhi, India

G. P. Rath (ed.), *Handbook of Trigeminal Neuralgia*,
https://doi.org/10.1007/978-981-13-2333-1_4

Classification

The two most commonly used classification systems are those proposed by the International Association for the Study of Pain (IASP) and the International Headache Society (IHS). According to the IASP classification, there are three subtypes of TGN: (1) Idiopathic, (2) Classical, and (3) Secondary. **Idiopathic TGN** denotes a condition of pain without any identifiable cause. In **Classical TGN**, there is vascular compression of the trigeminal nerve root resulting in morphological changes in the nerve. In **Secondary TGN**, the involvement of the trigeminal nerve is attributed to neurological diseases like tumors of the cerebellopontine angle or multiple sclerosis. In the classification system proposed by the IHS, TGN can be either: (1) Classical, or (2) Symptomatic [3, 4]. **Classical TGN (CTN)** is more common, and it is characterized by intermittent, severe, sharp, shooting, stabbing or electric shock-like pain lasting for a few seconds to minutes, with pain-free intervals between attacks. In most instances, the causative factor of CTN is compression of the trigeminal root by aberrant or tortuous vessels. **Symptomatic TGN (STN)**, on the other hand, is a variant predominated by constant aching, throbbing, or burning pain, with a minor component of sharp, episodes of pain. It is usually associated with a causative lesion, other than vascular compression, such as intracranial tumor, cholesteatoma, or multiple sclerosis.

Trigger Points/Zones

The pain in TGN is often initiated by triggering factors. It is usually triggered by some kind of tactile stimulus like talking, smiling, chewing, brushing or shaving to any area innervated by the trigeminal nerve. Some patients can pin-point these trigger areas on the face like cheek, lip or buccal mucosa. Presence of trigger zones is not a universal finding, but if present, they are pathognomonic of TGN [5]. Nearly half the patients of TGN experience a concomitant, continuous pain, also known as **background pain** [1]. Background pain can be aching, dull or burning in nature, and the intensity is usually of low severity. Background pain is more common in females. Patients with TGN also experience a "**refractory period**" after a paroxysmal attack, during which new attacks cannot be elicited. The exact pathophysiological basis of this refractory period is unknown but is postulated to be caused by hyperpolarization of the sensory neurons [1]. Like in many other chronic pain states, TGN can be associated with psychiatric problems, such as depression.

TGN is uncommon in young people. It is most often seen in adult females. A positive family history is found in a small proportion of patients. Patients with familial TGN can have bilateral distribution of pain [6]. In bilateral TGN, attacks are usually asynchronous, i.e. individual painful attacks are unilateral, with distinct episodes involving each side of the face at separate times [5, 6]. Patients with TGN tend to have stereotyped pain attacks, i.e. painful attacks are similar in nature and distribution in an individual patient. In case the nature or distribution of pain deviates markedly from the usual attacks, further investigations should be sought to exclude new neurological pathologies. Clinical presentations such as patients with bilateral symptoms, young patients, lack of triggered pain, absence of refractory period, abnormal neurological findings, pain outside the trigeminal nerve territory, presence of dizziness, vertigo or hearing loss, and visual disturbances should alarm the physician about the possibility of secondary TGN, and further investigations are warranted [7].

Diagnosis

TGN is a clinical diagnosis and physical examination is usually normal in patients with classical TGN. It is important to perform a thorough examination of the head and neck, with special attention to the ear, oral cavity, teeth and the temporomandibular joint. As discussed previously, presence of any sensory abnormality outside the trigeminal nerve territory, loss of corneal reflex, or facial muscle weakness warrants additional investigations to look for other causes. The diagnosis of TGN can be made when *at least three attacks* of unilateral facial pain occur, along with the following criteria (the International Classification of Headache Disorders, Third Edition):

1. Pain occurring in one or more divisions of the trigeminal nerve, with no radiation beyond the trigeminal distribution ***and***
2. Pain with ***at least three*** of the following four characteristics:
   (a) Recurring in paroxysmal attacks lasting from a fraction of a second to 2 min
   (b) Severe intensity
   (c) Electric shock-like, shooting, stabbing, or sharp in quality
   (d) Precipitated by innocuous stimuli to the affected side of the face

Although TGN may affect any branch of the trigeminal nerve, maxillary branch is most commonly affected, and ophthalmic branch is least commonly involved [8, 9]. Pain is usually right-sided, probably due to the narrower foramen rotundum and foramen ovale on the right side [5, 10].

According to the guidelines of the European Federation of Neurological Societies (EFNS) and the American Academy of Neurology (AAN), neurophysiological recording of the trigeminal reflexes is a reliable and useful test for neurophysiological diagnosis of TGN [11, 12]. This modality of diagnosis is however, not very common, and is supplanted by advanced neuroimaging tools.

Trigeminal Reflex Testing

It involves electrical stimulation of the divisions of the trigeminal nerve and measurement of the response with standard electromyography apparatus [9, 13]. The responses measured are V1-R1 (**blink reflex** after stimulation of supraorbital nerve), V2-SP1 (**masseter inhibitory reflex** after stimulation of infraorbital nerve) and

V3-SP1 (**masseter inhibitory reflex** after stimulation of mental nerve). The recordings are recorded externally from the orbicularis oculi muscle (for ophthalmic division) and the masseter muscle (for maxillary and mandibular divisions). Trigeminal reflex testing can be helpful to discover abnormalities in trigeminal nerve divisions that appear clinically unaffected. In patients with facial pain secondary to symptomatic TGN, post-herpetic neuralgia, vascular malformations, benign CPA tumors, or multiple sclerosis, an objective dysfunction is obtained with trigeminal reflex testing.

Imaging Studies

Apart from the clinical tests and the trigeminal reflexes, magnetic resonance imaging (MRI) has an important role in the diagnosis and treatment of TGN. The advancements in MR techniques have enabled precise diagnosis of the causes of symptomatic TGN [4, 9]. MRI of the brain should be performed in the initial evaluation of all patients presenting with signs and symptoms of TGN. When interpreting imaging scans, it is vital to understand that a single finding in the form of nerve-related changes or the presence of vascular compression, may not be always conclusive for the diagnosis of TGN. Imaging findings should always be interpreted in conjunction with clinical findings to decide further treatment strategies [14, 15].

Conclusion

Trigeminal neuralgia is a type of oro-facial pain with distinctive characteristics. The diagnosis is mostly based on clinical findings, but trigeminal reflex testing MRI sequences are important for confirming the diagnosis and finalizing the treatment plans.

References

1. Maarbjerg S, Di Stefano G, Bendtsen L, Cruccu G. Trigeminal neuralgia - diagnosis and treatment. Cephalalgia. 2017;37:648–57.
2. Headache Classification Committee of the International Headache Society (IHS). The international classification of headache disorders, 3rd edition (beta version). Cephalalgia. 2013;33:629–808.
3. Eller JL, Raslan AM, Burchiel KJ. Trigeminal neuralgia: definition and classification. Neurosurg Focus. 2005;18:E3.
4. Montano N, Conforti G, Di Bonaventura R, Meglio M, Fernandez E, Papacci F. Advances in diagnosis and treatment of trigeminal neuralgia. Ther Clin Risk Manag. 2015;11:289–99.
5. Neto HS, Camilli JA, Marques MJ. Trigeminal neuralgia is caused by maxillary and mandibular nerve entrapment: greater incidence of right-sided facial symptoms is due to the foramen rotundum and foramen ovale being narrower on the right side of the cranium. Med Hypotheses. 2005;65:1179–82.
6. Pollack IF, Jannetta PJ, Bissonette DJ. Bilateral trigeminal neuralgia: a 14-year experience with microvascular decompression. J Neurosurg. 1988;68:559–65.

7. Gronseth G, Cruccu G, Alksne J, Argoff C, Brainin M, Burchiel K, et al. Practice parameter: the diagnostic evaluation and treatment of trigeminal neuralgia (an evidence-based review): report of the Quality Standards Subcommittee of the American Academy of Neurology and the European Federation of Neurological Societies. Neurology. 2008;71:1183–90.
8. Katusic S, Beard CM, Bergstralh E, Kurland LT. Incidence and clinical features of trigeminal neuralgia, Rochester, Minnesota, 1945-1984. Ann Neurol. 1990;27:89–95.
9. Krafft RM. Trigeminal neuralgia. Am Fam Physician. 2008;77:1291–6.
10. Maarbjerg S, Gozalov A, Olesen J, Bendtsen L. Trigeminal neuralgia – a prospective systematic study of clinical characteristics in 158 patients. Headache. 2014;54:1574–82.
11. Cruccu G, Sommer C, Anand P, Attal N, Baron R, Garcia-Larrea L, et al. EFNS guidelines on neuropathic pain assessment: revised 2009. Eur J Neurol. 2010;17:1010–8.
12. Cruccu G, Gronseth G, Alksne J, Argoff C, Brainin M, Burchiel K, et al. AAN-EFNS guidelines on trigeminal neuralgia management. Eur J Neurol. 2008;15:1013–28.
13. Cruccu G, Finnerup NB, Jensen TS, Scholz J, Sindou M, Svensson P, et al. Trigeminal neuralgia: new classification and diagnostic grading for practice and research. Neurology. 2016;87:220–8.
14. Harsha KJ, Kesavadas C, Chinchure S, Thomas B, Jagtap S. Imaging of vascular causes of trigeminal neuralgia. J Neuroradiol. 2012;39:281–9.
15. Antonini G, Di Pasquale A, Cruccu G, Truini A, Morino S, Saltelli G, et al. Magnetic resonance imaging contribution for diagnosing symptomatic neurovascular contact in classical trigeminal neuralgia: a blinded case-control study and meta-analysis. Pain. 2014;155:1464–71.

Differential Diagnosis of Trigeminal Neuralgia

Deepa Dash

Key Points

- Trigeminal neuralgia (TGN) is characterized by incapacitating facial pain and its diagnosis is based mainly on history and clinical examination
- It is important to differentiate TGN from other disorders with facial pain for diagnostic precision and appropriate management
- Awareness on distinguishable clinical characteristics of other possible causes of facial pain such as dental problems, tempor-mandibular disorders, sinusitis, multiple sclerosis, neuralgias, and trigeminal autonomic cephalgias is necessary

Introduction

Trigeminal Neuralgia (TGN) is an important cause of facial pain and prevalence studies have shown that 0.07% of population may be afflicted with this disorder [1, 2]. The diagnosis of TGN is heavily dependent on clinical history provided by the patients. A detailed examination face and mouth helps ruling out different causes of facial pain. TGN is characterized by recurrent attacks of lancinating pain in the distribution of trigeminal nerve. The pain usually gets triggered by talking, chewing, brushing, shaving, a light touch or sometimes even a gentle breeze. It is unilateral most of the times and may occur repeatedly throughout the day. In classical TGN, no cause is identified other than neurovascular compression (NVC) whereas the symptomatic TGN may have an underlying cause. TGN may involve one or more branches of the trigeminal nerve, with the maxillary branch involved the

D. Dash (✉)
Department of Neurology, All India Institute of Medical Sciences (AIIMS), New Delhi, India

G. P. Rath (ed.), *Handbook of Trigeminal Neuralgia*,
https://doi.org/10.1007/978-981-13-2333-1_5

most often and the ophthalmic branch the least. The diagnosis is usually clinical, hence, the history of presentation is critical for the evaluation of these patients (Table 1).

Clinical Examination

Examination of a patient with facial pain should be comprehensive which starts from head and neck region and should include inspection of skin to observe for the changes in colorant abnormal swellings, and skin lesions. During the examination, salivary gland enlargement should be looked for. Examination should specifically focus on the muscles of mastication, head and neck for tenderness and trigger points, muscle hypertrophy, and movement of the temporo-mandibular joint (TMJ) including crepitus. The cranial nerves need to be examined. Intraoral examination includes the hard tissues and teeth for obvious dental pathology. The oral mucosa should be examined for soft tissue lesions. The differential diagnosis differs based on the duration and acuteness of the pain.

The clinical features are the red flags in a patient with classical TGN, and should raise doubts for secondary etiology or alternative diagnoses (Table 2). The following disorders will have to be kept in differential diagnosis of TGN.

Table 1 Information gathered on pain from the history

• Timing of pain, onset, duration, extent, severity, and periodicity
• Location and radiation
• Quality and severity
• Relieving and aggravating factors
• Any other special associated characteristics such as taste, salivary flow, clenching, bruxing habits, locking or clicking of jaw joint, altered sensation, nasal, eye or ear symptoms
• Presence of co-morbid pain conditions migraines, fibromyalgia
• Effect of pain on activities of daily living
• Co-morbid medical conditions
• History regarding psychological wellbeing of patient and stressors
• Drug history

Table 2 Red flags in patients with classic trigeminal neuralgia

• Sensory or motor deficits in cranial nerve examination
• Abnormal oral, dental, or ear examination
• Age younger than 40 years
• Presence of bilateral symptoms
• Dizziness or vertigo
• Hearing loss or abnormality
• Pain episodes persisting longer than two minutes
• Pain outside of trigeminal nerve distribution
• Visual findings

Dental Causes

The dental pain is usually unilateral and localized to mouth and hence could be confused with the pain of TGN. Diseases of the oral mucosa are very painful and are at times associated with a lesion. The pain is continuous in nature and not of paroxysmal type described for TGN. A detailed examination of the teeth, gingiva, and oral mucosa may help identifying the cause.

Temporo-Mandibular Disorders (TMD)

One of the commonest differentials for patients presenting with acute facial pain is the disorders affecting the temporo-mandibular joint (TMJ). TMD has been reported in 5–12% of general population with usual age of affliction at 20–40 years [3]. Pain in these conditions is usually encountered when the opening of mouth is prolonged. Muscles of mastication and neck are most commonly affected; local examination would provide further clues on the diagnosis of TMD. When the joint is palpated, the patient may appreciate similar pain characteristics. Clicks are seen when patients have intra-articular disc diseases and there may be locking if the disc does not reduce on its own. Crepitus may be detected in patients with degenerative disorders of TMJ. Subluxation problems are mainly found in patients with hypermobility and are associated with deviation of jaws on mouth opening. Imaging (e.g. X-ray) is not required for masticatory problems but can be useful in joint disorders, although its current role is controversial [4].

Disorders of Salivary Glands

Disorders that affect drainage of the salivary glands due to various etiology such as tumors, mechanical obstruction and subsequent infection may present with pain along distribution of the trigeminal nerve. Salivary gland duct blockage can be due to formation of stones. This type of pain presents before eating and is of intermittent in nature. Diagnosis is supported by the palpation of the stone; the salivary flow may be slow or absent. Imaging and ultrasound can help clinching the diagnosis.

Maxillary Sinusitis

The pain due to maxillary sinusitis is usually encountered in acute settings; the chronic form is less likely to be associated with pain. On examination, tenderness is elicited over the maxillary sinus which is a clue for the diagnosis. The nature of pain is mild-to-moderate dull, continuous, aching, boring type and gets aggravated on bending. A history of nasal discharge, respiratory infection, or dental treatment is associated with the maxillary sinusitis.

Trigeminal Autonomic Cephalalgias (TACs)

The TACs constitute a group of primary headache disorders characterized by cranial autonomic symptoms and pain in the territory of trigeminal nerve innervation. The disorders included cluster headache, paroxysmal hemicranias, short-lasting unilateral neuralgiform headache attacks with conjuctival injection and tearing (SUNCT), short lasting unilateral neuralgiform headache attacks with cranial autonomic symptoms (SUNA) and hemicrania continua (Table 3).

The location of pain may be a useful distinguishing feature between TGN and TAC. Pain in TGN is confined to the trigeminal sensory distribution, more commonly in the maxillary (V2) (35%) and mandibular distribution (V3) (30%) compared to the ophthalmic distribution (V1) (10%) [5]. In SUNCT pain is more common in V1 (67%) and V2 (33%), and is very unlikely in V3. In SUNA, 56% of patients report pain in V1, 56% in V2, and 33% in V3 [6]. The strict confinement to trigeminal sensory distribution is not seen in SUNCT and SUNA. The duration of pain also helps in differentiating the three; a shorter-duration attack may be seen in TGN compared to SUNCT/SUNA. Various patterns of pain have been described with SUNCT/SUNA syndrome. The autonomic symptoms are usually intense and may present as conjuctival injection, lacrimation, nasal congestion, rhinorrhoea, edema of eyelids, sweating and flushing of forehead and face, sensation of fullness in ear, ptosis or miosis [7]. In contrast to the TACs, TGN is rarely associated with autonomic symptoms. In a study by Simms on 92 patients who underwent surgical procedure for TGN, 67% of patients had at least one autonomic symptom and 14% had four or more symptoms [8]. With V1 pain, the most common symptoms were ptosis, lacrimation and conjuctival injection whereas with V2 involvement it was facial swelling. Triggering factors are not only seen in TGN but also in SUNCT and SUNA patients; they are more in SUNCT than SUNA. Presence of a refractory

Table 3 Differentiating features between trigeminal neuralgia and short-lasting unilateral neuralgiform headaches

Parameters	Trigeminal neuralgia	SUNCT/SUNA
Gender predisposition	Female predominant	Male predominant: SUNCT Female predominant: SUNA
Pain distribution	Trigeminal nerve distribution only	Pain outside the trigeminal territory
Duration of attacks	Less than 10 s	Range: 240–600 s
Intensity of autonomic symptoms	Mild	Severe
Refractory period	Present	No refractory period
Responsiveness to carbamazepine	Maximum	Less

SUNCT Short-lasting unilateral neuralgiform headache attacks with conjuctival injection and tearing, *SUNA* Short lasting unilateral neuralgiform headache attacks with cranial autonomic symptoms

period is seen in TGN, but, not in SUNCT/SUNA. Response to carbamazepine therapy helps in differentiating TGN from SUNCT or SUNA. Reduction of pain is seen in 80% of patients to a trial of carbamazepine therapy whereas it may be observed in 39% of SUNCT and 20% of SUNA cases [9].

Cluster Headache

Cluster headache is usually seen in late third or early fourth decade. There is a temporal association of headache with sleep; it usually starts approximately 90 min after the patient falls asleep. The pain is episodic, always unilateral, typically periorbital, and with a relatively prolonged course which may last for 15–180 min. The pain is usually not preceded by an aura and is of constant, severe, throbbing, and stabbing type. The patients may present with signs of Horner's syndrome and conjuctival injection when examined at the time of an attack; it helps diagnosing the condition.

Glossopharyngeal Neuralgia

Glossopharyngeal neuralgia (GPN) is a rare condition as compared to TGN, occurs due to hyperactivity of glossopharyngeal nerve. The pain is unilateral in distribution with involvement of ear, tongue, and areas inferior to the angle of the mandible. The paroxysmal attacks usually last from seconds to minutes, and usually recur multiple times a day and may remit in between for weeks to months. The pain is characterized by sharp, shooting, electric shock-like sensations in the posterior part of throat, base of tongue, tonsillar fossa, ear canal, and areas inferior to angle of mandible. It is usually presented in a female as a painful condition on left side unlike TGN which is more common on right side. It is precipitated by swallowing, chewing, coughing, yawning, talking, and swallowing. Anticonvulsants like carbamazepine, gabapentin, and pregabalin remains first-line of treatment. Some patients may have their symptoms under satisfactory control with medical therapy, but, in many patients pain may become refractory to medication or require increasing doses, over period of time.

Post-herpetic Neuralgia (PHN)

PHN is characterized by history of mucocutaneous involvement by herpes zoster (HZ) and pain in the dermatomal distribution of the vesico-papular rash. The pain usually starts weeks to months after the resolution of manifestations of HZ. It is characterized by allodynia and pain which may be described as burning, sharp, shooting, or electric shock-like types. Within the affected dermatomes, there may be areas of diminution of sensations of vibration, pinprick, or heat. The pain is continuous in nature with fluctuations in the severity and character.

Nervus Intermedius Neuralgia

Similar to TGN, nervus intermedius neuralgia is also associated with brief, paroxysmal pain but the location is usually in the depths of ear. The trigger zone is different from TGN and is the posterior wall of the auricular canal. The character of pain is similar to that encountered in TGN and also may radiate to the parietal-occipital region or to trigeminal sensory zones.

Tic Convulsif and Hemifacial Spasm

The disease is characterized by co-existent TGN and hemifacial spasm. It is usually caused by neurovascular compression in posterior fossa. It can be differentiated by the presence of the involuntary contraction of facial muscles on one side.

Tolosa-Hunt Syndrome

Tolosa-Hunt syndrome is a disease characterized by painful opthalmoplegia and nonspecific inflammation of the cavernous sinus or superior orbital fissure. The major differentiating feature is the presence of cranial nerve deficit in this syndrome. The third, fourth, and fifth cranial nerves are commonly affected. The pain usually precedes the opthalmoparesis but presence of the cranial nerve deficits will help differentiate it from TGN.

Multiple Sclerosis (MS)

MS is an auto-immune and demyelinating disease which affects the brain and spinal cord causing wide range of symptoms like problems with vision, limb movement, and sensation or balance. Presence of bilateral TGN suggests a possible association with MS. Pathophysiologically, MS is characterized by demyelination of primary sensory trigeminal afferents in the root entry zone. Patients with MS are much more likely to develop TGN than patients without MS; these patients are young in age. The diagnosis of MS usually precedes the presentation of TGN.

Conclusion

It is very import to take a detailed history covering all important aspects while assessing a patient with short-lasting unilateral facial pain. Supportive clinical features such as the gender of patient; severity, localization, and duration of pain; intensity and natural history of autonomic symptoms; refractoriness; and the response to treatment may help distinguishing the conditions. Classification using all potentially distinguishable clinical characteristics may improve the diagnostic precision leading to appropriate treatment and improved outcome.

References

1. Macfarlane TV, Beasley M, Macfarlane GJ. Self-reported facial pain in UK biobank study: prevalence and associated factors. J Oral Maxillofac Res. 2014;5:e2.
2. van Hecke O, Austin SK, Khan RA, et al. Neuropathic pain in the general population: a systematic review of epidemiological studies. Pain. 2014;155:654–62.
3. Fillingim RB, Slade GD, Diatchenko L, et al. Summary of findings from the OPPERA baseline case-control study: implications and future directions. J Pain. 2011;12:T102–7.
4. Petersson A. What you can and cannot see in TMJ imaging — an overview related to the RDC/TMD diagnostic system. J Oral Rehabil. 2010;37:771–8.
5. Lambru G, Matharu MS. SUNCT, SUNA and trigeminal neuralgia: different disorders or variants of the same disorder? Curr Opin Neurol. 2014;27:325–31.
6. Cohen AS, Matharu MS, Goadsby PJ. Short-lasting unilateral neuralgiform headache attacks with conjunctival injection and tearing (SUNCT) or cranial autonomic features (SUNA)-a prospective clinical study of SUNCT and SUNA. Brain. 2006;129:2746–60.
7. Headache Classification Subcommittee of the International Headache Society. The International Classification of Headache Disorders, 3rd edn. Cephalalgia. 2013;33:629–808.
8. Simms HN, Honey CR. The importance of autonomic symptoms in trigeminal neuralgia. Clinical article. J Neurosurg. 2011;115:210–6.
9. Cohen AS. Short-lasting unilateral neuralgiform headache attacks with conjunctival injection and tearing. Cephalalgia. 2007;27:824–32.

Therapeutic Options for Trigeminal Neuralgia

Charu Mahajan

Key Points

- The choice of therapeutic modality in patients with trigeminal neuralgia (TGN) depends upon etiopathogenesis, clinical presentation, age, and associated comorbidities
- Pain in TGN recurs and effectiveness of major therapeutic modalities wanes over time; utility of multimodal approach comes into play in such scenario
- Apart from resolving sensory symptoms, a holistic approach is required for overall social, emotional, and neuropsychological rehabilitation of the patient
- A stepwise algorithm for management of TGN has been proposed

Introduction

The trigeminal neuralgia (TGN) is an immensely painful entity which often compromises the quality of life. Recurrent paroxysms over course of time become resistant to treatment resulting in a chronic pain syndrome which affects psychological and cognitive domain causing anxiety and depression. This chapter highlights the overview of various therapeutic options along with multimodal management of TGN.

C. Mahajan (✉)
Department of Neuroanaesthesiology and Critical Care, All India Institute of Medical Sciences (AIIMS), New Delhi, India

G. P. Rath (ed.), *Handbook of Trigeminal Neuralgia*,
https://doi.org/10.1007/978-981-13-2333-1_6

Choice of Treatment

The choice of therapeutic modality for treatment of TGN is guided by etiology, pathophysiology, clinical presentation, age, and co-morbidities. The atypical trigeminal neuralgic pain requires treatment of the underlying conditions such as tumors, multiple sclerosis (MS), post-herpetic and post-surgical conditions. Oral pharmacotherapy is usually the first line of management [1]. The antiepileptic drugs such as carbamazepine (CBZ) and oxcarbamazepine (OXZ) remain the first line drugs of choice. Although evidence is stronger for CBZ, but the OXZ has lesser side effects, albeit with almost similar efficacy. If initiation of treatment, in daily doses is not effective, the dose is either escalated or add-on therapy with second-line drugs ensued. These include lamotrigine and baclofen, both of which decrease the excitatory neurotransmission. Inadequate control of pain may lead to addition of another third line of drugs which include alternative options like phenytoin, gabapentin, pregabalin, levetiracetam, valproate, clonazepam, and topiramate.

Patients refractory to medical treatment (not relieved by an adequate trial of at least three drugs in sufficient dosage) are the candidates for next step of management i.e. surgical intervention. These may be invasive [microvascular decompression (MVD) of trigeminal nerve], minimally invasive [percutaneous rhizotomy] or non-invasive modalities [stereotactic radiosurgery by gamma knife or cybersurgery] depending upon the nature of procedure performed.

Another way of classification of the management strategy is based on the site of intervention, as below.

1. **Subdermal Therapies** involve either subcutaneous lignocaine or alcohol blockade of specific branch of trigeminal nerve. Botulinum neurotoxin (BoNT) type A produces analgesic effect in neuropathic pain and can be administered intradermally or submucosally [2].
2. **Peripheral Percutaneous Techniques** incorporate the use of chemical (alcohol, phenol, and glycerol) or thermal energy (radiofrequency ablation) to produce a lesion in the branches distal to the Gasserian ganglion. Other less popular techniques are peripheral cryotherapy (performed by surgically exposing the nerve intraorally) and peripheral injection of streptomycin-lidocaine.
3. **Percutaneous Techniques on Gasserian Ganglion** destroy the nerve fibers by employing either radiofrequency, chemicals (glycerol) or mechanical force (percutaneous balloon compression)
4. **Posterior Fossa Procedures** can be invasive or non-invasive.

   (a) **Invasive Procedures**

   - **Microvascular Decompression (MVD) of trigeminal nerve**: It is the procedure of choice for classic TGN with neurovascular compression or conflict (NVC). At the level of the posterior fossa, open surgical technique involves the correction of NVC by separation of vessel and nerve, and keeping them apart. The reported success rate of MVD is as high as 83.5% (80–89%) with a severe complication rate of 0.1% [3].

- **Partial Sensory Rhizotomy (PSR)**: In those patients without NVC or presence of inoperable vascular anatomy and in those with relapsing pain after MVD, destructive procedures such as PSR may be considered as an alternative. However, PSR is rarely performed these days.
- **Internal Neurolysis** is another surgical alternative where nerve fibers are separated longitudinally causing lesser damage to nerve as compared to PSR, thus resulting in lesser sensory deficits [4].
- **Cryotherapy** involves frozen application at particular branch of the nerve after it has been surgically exposed [5].

(b) **Non-invasive Procedure**

- **Stereotactic Radiosurgery (SRS)** is another ablative non-invasive procedure by means of gamma knife (GK) therapy wherein irradiation of nerve causes an electric block of pain transmission. The more recent cybersurgery involves frameless stereotaxy. The drawback of GK is onset of pain relief which may take several weeks to 2–3 months. If performed as a primary treatment, it has a better prognosis rather than when attempted after surgical intervention [6]. However, it can be done as a repeat procedure even if it fails during first time, but with a lower success rate.
- **Low-level Laser therapy** uses a single wavelength light which alters cell and tissue function. In many studies, it has been found to decrease intensity and frequency of pain without any side effects [7].

These above procedures are effective to a variable rate depending upon the etiopathogenesis of typical TGN.

Atypical TGN is characterized by constant neuropathic type of pain secondary to trauma, surgery, post-herpes or MS. In these cases, pain is often resistant to medical management and standard therapies are ineffectual. Percutaneous techniques and SRS are the preferred modalities of treatment. Neuromodulation procedures (Table 1) alter the nerve activity through targeted delivery of a stimulus either electrical or chemical to trigeminal nerve, peripheral nerves, motor cortex or spinal cord. These procedures may be classified as invasive or non-invasive and central or peripheral as below.

Table 1 Neuromodulation Procedures for Trigeminal Neuralgia

Invasive Procedures
• Transcutaneous Electrical Pulsed Stimulation Of Trigeminal Nerve/ Peripheral Nerve Stimulation (Supraorbital, infraorbital, occipital)
• Gasserian Ganglion Pulsed Stimulation
• Motor Cortex Stimulation
• Deep Brain Stimulation
• Spinal Cord Stimulation
• Sphenopalatine Ganglion Blockade
Non-invasive Procedures
• Transcranial Magnetic Stimulation
• Transcranial Direct Current Stimulation
• Transcutaneous Electrical Nerve Stimulation (TENS)

1. **Peripheral Nerve Stimulation** (Supraorbital, infraorbital, occipital): Subcutaneous electrodes are placed in the nerve distribution which are connected to an implanted pulse generator. Peripheral nerve field stimulation is a variant of this technique where electrodes are placed in the region of pain instead of particular nerve.
2. **Trigeminal Ganglion Stimulation** involves percutaneous placement of an electrode in postganglionic trigeminal nerve followed by test stimulation. After successful pain relief, an electrode pulse generator system is implanted.
3. **Motor Cortex Stimulation**: A small craniotomy is used for placement of electrode grid on the motor cortex opposite to the painful side, followed by lead tunneling and exteriorization. The leads are connected to an external stimulus generator for testing for optimum stimulation intensity for pain relief. If patients experience satisfactory pain relief, the electrodes are connected to an implantable pulse generator which is placed subcutaneously.
4. **Deep Brain Stimulation**: Under stereotactic guidance, electrodes are placed in ventral posterior thalamus and periaqueductal gray/periventricular gray matter. After a phase of trial stimulation and adequate pain relief, electrode leads are internalized and a subcutaneous pulse generator is implanted.
5. **Spinal Cord Stimulation**: Electrodes are surgically implanted at cervicomedullary junction and connected to an external pulse generator placed in subclavicular area. Spinal cord is thus stimulated via low intensity electric impulses, which creates a neuromodulatory effect on the nervous system.
6. **Transcranial Magnetic Stimulation**: In this technique, cortical neurons in primary motor cortex are non-invasively stimulated using transcranial magnetic stimulation pulses. The M1 projections to pain modulating structures like medial thalamus and periaqueductal gray matter produces pain relief.
7. **Transcutaneous Electrical Nerve Stimulation (TENS)**: The external patch electrodes are placed in the region of the affected nerve. External pulse generator applies pulsed electrical stimulation which can be modified in terms of rate, intensity, and duration of stimulation.

These techniques have been described in various case series but evidence is not strong enough to incorporate them in routine treatment [8]. They need to be evaluated further by randomized control trials which would validate their role and effectiveness.

A stepwise algorithm for management of TGN is depicted in Fig. 1. After the clinical diagnosis is made, the first step is to provide medical management. If MRI confirms the presence of neurovascular conflict (NVC), age and presence of other co-morbidities are taken into consideration while deciding the management options. MVD has a higher long-term efficacy and thus, patients who are young without any comorbidities, tolerate this open surgical procedure well. In patients who do not have NVC, the role of MVD is unclear. In these operated patients, if recurrence of TGN occurs early, it may be taken as an inadequately performed procedure and a second attempt at MVD is justified. In case the pain recurs late, other modalities of treatment are such as percutaneous techniques or SRS are tried. Percutaneous rhizotomy techniques are useful in patients with age more than 75 years who is not fit

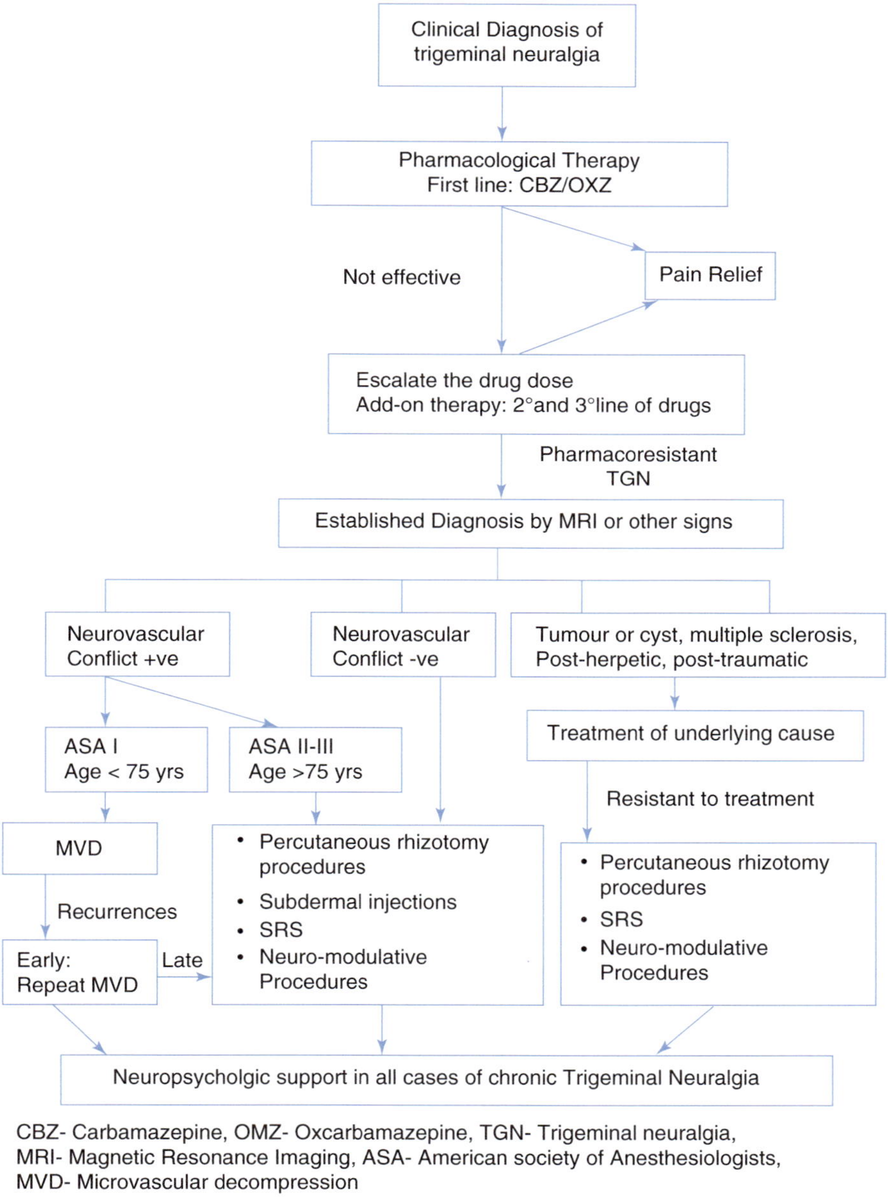

Fig. 1 Algorithm Depicting the Step-Wise Approach to Trigeminal Neuralgia.

to undergo a major neurosurgical procedure, or if there is absence of NVC. Radiofrequency ablation is the favored technique amongst all percutaneous procedures. Although these procedures are minimally invasive, the pain relief may not last for long. Non-invasive SRS with GK is helpful in patients not fit for surgery or in those in whom NVC is absent. For atypical TGN, percutaneous rhizotomy procedures and SRS are the treatment options. However, for the pain resistant to all these modalities neuromodulation procedures may be tried.

TGN may be difficult to treat and recurrent attacks may lead to a more protracted chronic course affecting the neuropsychology and cognition of the patient. Patient may experience anxiety, depression, mood disorders, somatic misperception of pain, dysfunction of memory and cognitive function overall. Thus, along with the therapeutic management of pain, neuropsychologic evaluation and support are a very important component of comprehensive treatment.

Conclusion

The therapeutic modalities aim to control the trigeminal pain at various levels from its origin in the posterior fossa, at gasserian ganglion, to its terminal branches. No single drug or technique is completely effective in abolishing the pain. All these therapies have an effect which is not permanent and pain recurrence rates are high and variable depending upon the technique chosen. Thus, majority of the patients require a multi-modal approach for control of pain due to trigeminal neuralgia.

References

1. Gronseth G, Cruccu G, Alksne J, Argoff C, Brainin M, Burchiel K, Nurmikko T, Zakrzewska JM. Practice parameter: the diagnostic evaluation and treatment of trigeminal neuralgia (an evidence-based review): report of the Quality Standards Subcommittee of the American Academy of Neurology and the European Federation of Neurological Societies. Neurology. 2008;71:1183–90.
2. Wu CJ, Lian YJ, Zheng YK, Zhang HF, Chen Y, Xie NC, Wang LJ. Botulinum toxin type A for the treatment of trigeminal neuralgia: results from a randomized, double-blind, placebo-controlled trial. Cephalalgia. 2012;32:443–50.
3. Xia L, Zhong J, Zhu J, Wang YN, Dou NN, Liu MX, Visocchi M, Li ST. Effectiveness and safety of microvascular decompression surgery for treatment of trigeminal neuralgia: a systematic review. J Craniofac surg 2014;25:1413-7.
4. Ko AL, Lee A, Raslan AM, Ozpinar A, MCCartney S, Burchiel KJ. Long term efficacy and safety of internal neurolysis for trigeminal neuralgia without neurovascular compression. J Neurosurg. 2015;122:1048–57.
5. Toda K. Operative treatment of trigeminal neuralgia: review of current techniques. Oral Surg Oral Med Oral Pathol Oral Radiol Endod. 2008;106:788–805.
6. Wolf A, Kondziolka D. Gamma knife surgery in trigeminal neuralgia. Neurosurg Clin N Am. 2016;27:297–304.
7. Falaki F, Nejat AH, Dalirsani Z. The effect of low-level laser therapy on trigeminal neuralgia: a review of literature. J Dent Res Dent Clin Dent Prospects. 2014;8:1–5.
8. Weber K. Neuromodulation and devices in trigeminal neuralgia. Headache. 2017;57:1648–53.

Radiology for Trigeminal Neuralgia

Pankaj Surange, Harshita Surange, and Gaurav Goyal

Key Points

- The diagnosis of trigeminal neuralgia (TGN) is mainly clinical, but radiological imaging helps understanding etio-pathogeneis and hence, for subsequent management
- Magnetic resonance imaging (MRI) is the mainstay of diagnosis as it reveals fine anatomic details and helps analyzing the entire course of the trigeminal nerve
- Interventional treatment of patient (three-dimensional) is usually based on fluoroscopic images (two-dimensional)
- The success of percutaneous surgical procedures requires a thorough understanding of radiologic anatomy of base and lateral views of the skull

Introduction

The diagnosis of trigeminal neuralgia (TGN) is mainly based on patient's history and clinical examination. Classically, the patient presents with characteristic paroxysm of pain, with short and severe episodes, which is typically unilateral, and along the course of the trigeminal nerve. There is a greater predilection towards the right side.

P. Surange (✉)
World Institute of Pain (India Chapter), New Delhi, India

Interventional Pain and Spine Centre (IPSC), New Delhi, India

H. Surange
Diagnostic and Imaging Centre, New Delhi, India

G. Goyal
Interventional Pain and Spine Centre (IPSC), New Delhi, India

G. P. Rath (ed.), *Handbook of Trigeminal Neuralgia*,
https://doi.org/10.1007/978-981-13-2333-1_7

Apart from the idiopathic variety, secondary causes of TGN must be ruled out, as neuropathy of trigeminal nerve may involve the nerve anywhere along its course, from the nerve nuclei to the peripheral branches. Since clinical findings alone are not sufficient to localize the site of the causative lesion, magnetic resonance imaging (MRI) must be carried out before any intervention is planned. Imaging may also help to diagnose an enlarged loop of artery or vein compressing the trigeminal nerve, i.e. neurovascular compression (NVC) at the cerebellopontine (CP) angle, plaques in multiple sclerosis (MS), and tumor in the CP angle region. A thorough understanding of the x-ray anatomy of base and lateral view of the skull is important, as majority of the interventions are performed with fluoroscopic-guided techniques. This chapter covers the diagnostic and therapeutic aspects of radiology in patients of TGN.

Diagnostic Radiology for Trigeminal Neuralgia

MRI for Trigeminal Nerve and Ganglion

MRI is the imaging modality of choice to visualize the entire course of the trigeminal nerve [1]. The nerve has four nuclei (a) mesencephalic nucleus, which mediates proprioception, (b) sensory nucleus for tactile sensation, (c) motor nucleus for motor innervation, and (d) spinal nucleus, which mediates pain and temperature. The nerve root enters the Meckel's cave into the cerebrospinal fluid (CSF) filled subarachnoid space known as the *trigeminal cistern.* It then forms a ganglion known as the *trigeminal or Gasserian ganglion*, which is the site of deposition of agents for chemical neurolysis. Distal to the Gasserian ganglion, the nerve trifurcates into ophthalmic (V1), maxillary (V2), and mandibular (V3) nerves.

The trigeminal nerve fibers originate from the grey matter nuclei present in the brainstem and the first spinal cervical segment. The fibers from all these nuclei converge and emerge from the anterolateral aspect of the pons. It is a mixed nerve with a thick lateral sensory and a thin medial motor root (Fig. 1). The course of the trigeminal nerve can be divided into: (a) intra-axial segment, (b) cisternal component, (c) Gasserian ganglion in the Meckel's cave, (d) cavernous segment, and (e) extra-cranial component [2]. Brain stem pathologies like infarct, glioma, and MS are common causes involving the intra-axial segment of the nerve [3]. Neurovascular compression (NVC) is the commonest cause for cisternal component involvement (Fig. 2) followed by trigeminal schwannoma (Fig. 3), meningioma, arachnoid and epidermoid cysts, and infective pathologies (Fig. 4). Gasserian ganglion and cavernous segments can be involved in

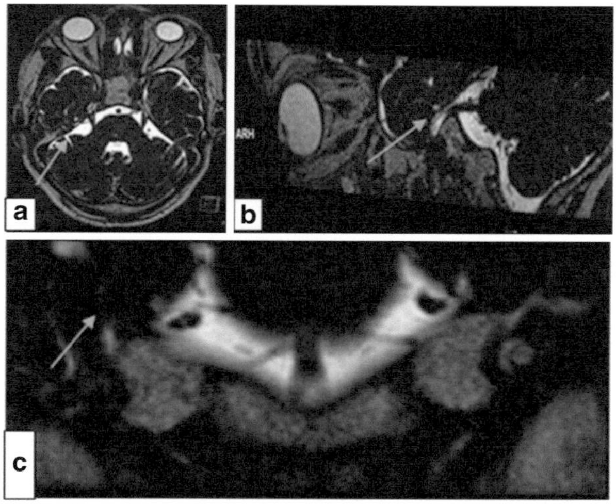

Fig. 1 Three-dimensional sampling perfection with application-optimized contrast using different flip-angle (3D-SPACE) axial sagittal (**a**), oblique (**b**), and coronal (**c**) views showing normal anatomy of the cisternal segment of trigeminal nerve (short arrow points to the motor and the long arrow points to sensory root)

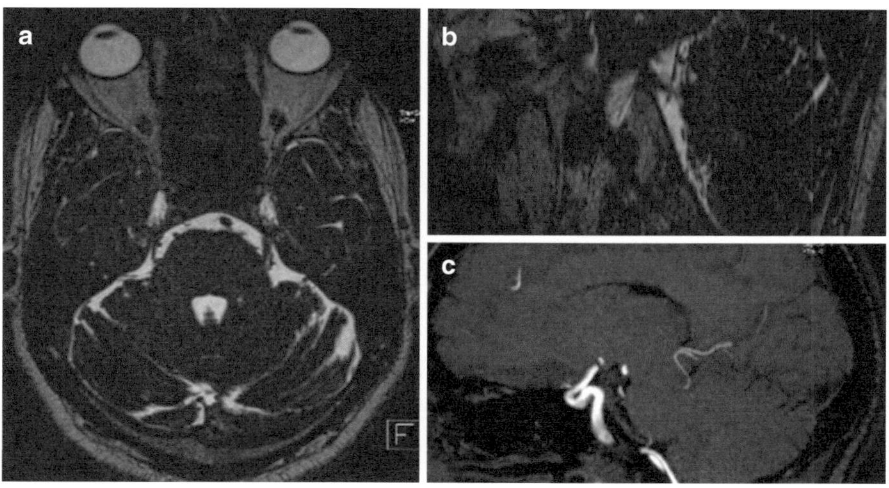

Fig. 2 Axial SPACE image showing atrophy of the cisternal component of right trigeminal nerve (**a**); sagittal SPACE image showing superior cerebellar artery (SCA) crossing the TZ of the cisternal part of trigeminal nerve resulting in atrophy (**b**); MIP TOF sagittal oblique image showing contact of the SCA with the trigeminal nerve (**c**) in a patient with trigeminal neuralgia in right side

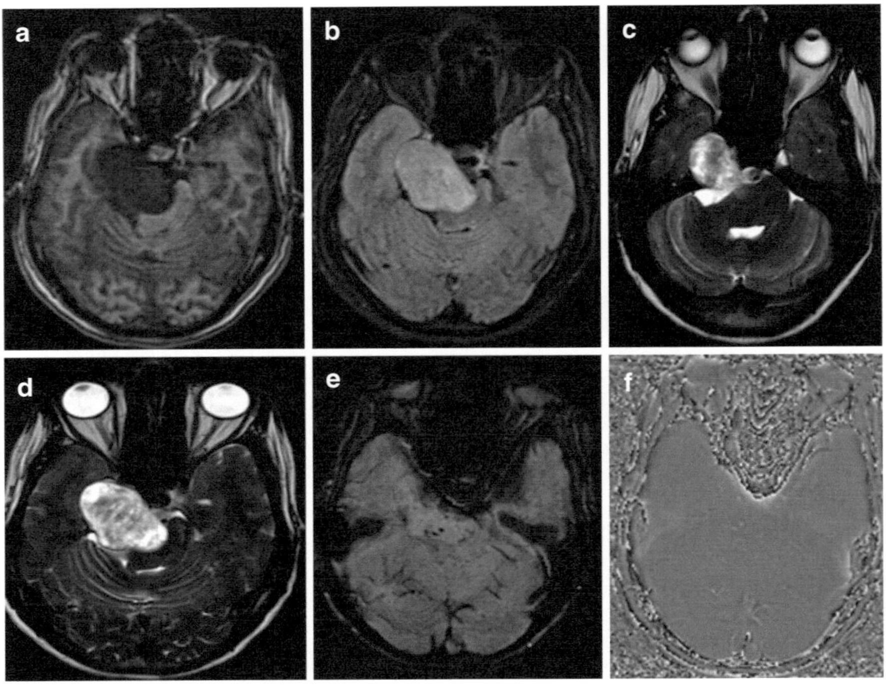

Fig. 3 MRI brain shows trigeminal schwannoma which is isointense on T1 (**a**) and FLAIR (**b**) sequences and is heterogeneously hyperintense on T2 (**c**, **d**) sequences. SWI images (**e**, **f**) showing petechial hemorrhages in the trigeminal schwannoma in a patient with right trigeminal neuralgia

meningioma, schwannoma (Fig. 5) hemangioma, aneurysms and intracranial metastasis. Perineural tumor spread most commonly involves the extracranial part of the trigeminal nerve [4].

The first successful use of MRI for detection of NVC was reported by Tash and colleagues in 1989 [5]. MRI for TGN should include the basic standard brain sequences along with advanced pulse sequences to delineate various pathologies in detail (Table 1). ***CISS (Constructive Interference in Steady State)*** is a part of fast gradient echo sequences and considered to be superior to the conventional plain MRI [6]. It has advantages of high spatial resolution and contrast between the structures and allows for the detailed study of trigeminal nerve. Introduction of 3D-CISS

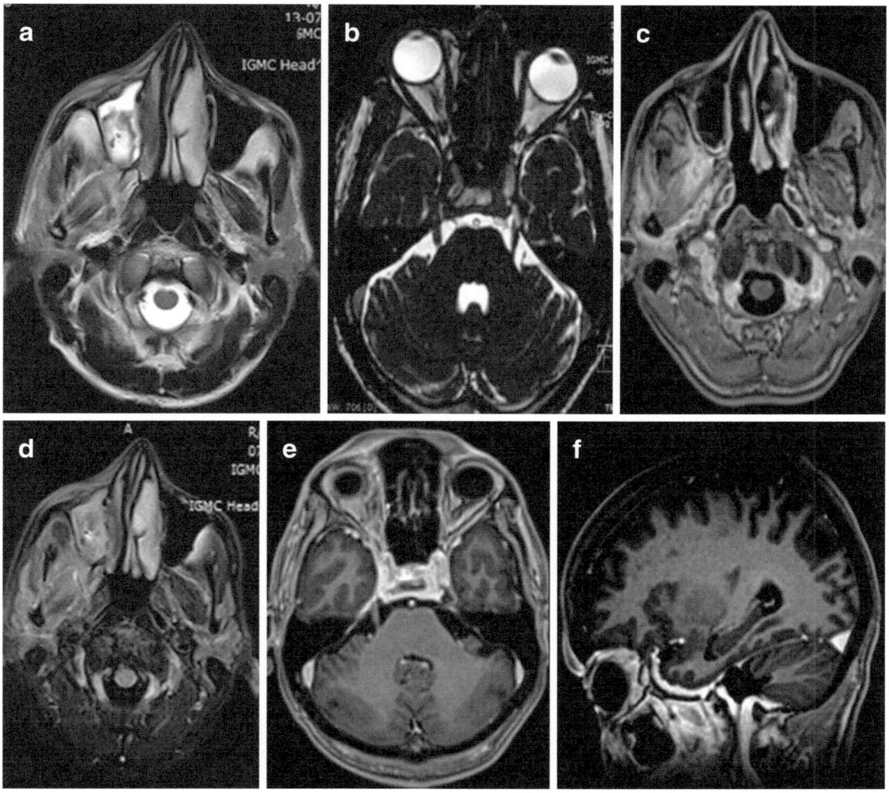

Fig. 4 T2-weighted axial sequence showing right maxillary sinusitis with heterogenous hyperintensity in the muscles of masticator space and infratemporal fossa in right side (**a**); axial SPACE sequence showing thickened right trigeminal nerve (**b**); axial post-contrast sequences showing enhancement in the right-sided muscles of the masticator space, infratemporal fossa, and maxillary sinus (**c**, **d**); axial and sagittal post-contrast sequences (**e**, **f**) showing enhancing cisternal segment of right trigeminal nerve and thick, continuous, nodular enhancement of the pachymeninges along the antero-inferior surface of right temporal lobe in a patient with right trigeminal pain

helped detailed visualization of NVC and plays a significant role in searching for vascular compression [7]. Apart from diagnosing the etiology, it also helps in determining the extent of NVC [8]. CISS is a modification of the conventional MRI and

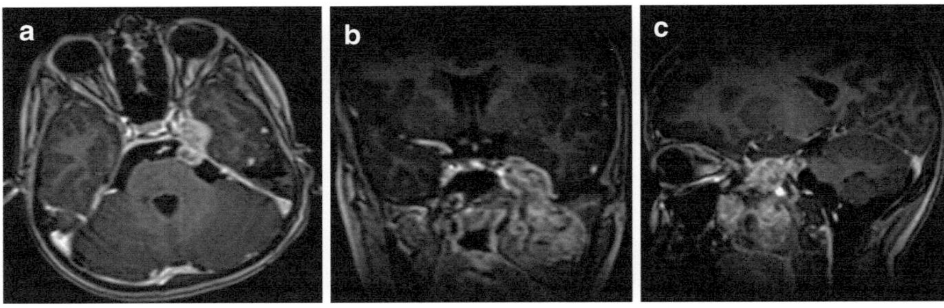

Fig. 5 Post-contrast axial images shows trigeminal nerve schwannoma involving the cisternal and the cavernous component giving rise to dumbell shape (**a**); coronal image shows cavernous component of trigeminal schwannoma extending into the masticator space through foramen ovale (**b**); sagittal image shows extension of intracranial trigeminal schwannoma in masticator space and infratemporal fossa through the foramen ovale (**c**) in a patient with left trigeminal neuralgia

Table 1 Advanced magnetic resonance imaging MRI protocols for diagnosis of trigeminal neuralgia [13, 20]

Protocol (s)	Benefit (s)
Whole brain 3D T1-weighted fast spoiled gradient recalled pulse sequence	Provides excellent tissue contrast and high spatial resolution
Whole brain axial T2 weighted sequence	Delineates pathologies
Whole brain axial FLAIR sequence	Better delineation of pathologies
Heavily T2-weighted thin section multiplanar SSFP sequence through the brain stem	Delineates entire cisternal portion of the nerve along with Gasserian ganglion
3D-TOF MR angiography for circle of Willis	Carried out when NVC is suspected
Post-contrast whole brain 3D T1-weighted fast spoiled gradient recalled pulse sequence after contrast administration	Optional; when a space occupying or inflammatory pathology is suspected

3D Three dimensional, *SSFP* Steady state free precession, *3D-TOF* Three-dimensional time-of-flight, *MR* Magnetic resonance, *FLAIR* Fluid attenuated inversion recovery, *NVC* Neurovascular compression

is available in MR machine with strength higher than 1.5 Tesla. Different names are used by different manufacturers (Table 2) [6].

Recently, high-resolution *diffusion tensor imaging (DTI) with trigeminal tractography* has been used [9] for detection of microstructure changes to the trigeminal nerve in patients with TGN. To add to the diagnosis of NVC, fusion imaging involving the steady state free precession (SSFP) sequence, and 3D-TOF magnetic resonance (MR) angiography can be done for better visualization of nerve compression by the artery [10].

The trigeminal nerve carries myelin sheath along its course; oligodendrocytes form the myelin in the central nervous system (CNS) and Schwann cells form the myelin in peripheral nervous system (PNS). *Transition zone (TZ) or Redlich-Obersteiner's zone*, also known as the root entry zone (REZ), is the portion of the nerve at the junction of the central and peripheral myelin [11]. TZ is vulnerable to mechanical stresses, as central myelin is thinner than peripheral myelin, and it is less-capable of repair following damage. In trigeminal nerve, the maximum length of centrally myelinated segment is about 48% of the total cisternal component [11]. Root entry/exit zone is defined as the portion of the nerve that includes TZ, central myelin portion, and adjacent brain stem surface [12].

Most TGNs are idiopathic; however, among the secondary causes, NVC is an important differential, and MRI plays a key role in its diagnosis. Superior cerebellar artery (SCA), anterior inferior cerebellar artery (AICA), vertebrobasilar dolichoectasia or venous compressions are the main causes of nerve compression in the cisternal segment. Proximal vascular compression of the cisternal segment is considered clinically more relevant than the distal compression. Not all the vascular compressions of the nerve are clinically significant, as prevalence of asymptomatic vascular contact is also very high. Hence, clinical-radiological correlation is considered to be essential. Radiologically, diagnostic signs such as loss of intervening cerebrospinal fluid (CSF) between nerve and vessel, nerve displacement by the vessel, and atrophy of the nerve in the TZ due to focal demyelination are helpful in diagnosing NVC syndrome [13]. The extent of compression of the nerve and vessel has been graded based on MRI (Table 3) [12]. In patients with Grade 3 NVC, thinning and atrophy of trigeminal nerve renders them refractory to medications, with possible need for surgical interventions.

Table 2 Different names of CISS sequence by various manufacturers [6]

Different Names of CISS Sequence	Manufacturer
Fast Imaging Employing Steady-state Acquisition (FIESTA)	GE Healthcare
True Fast Imaging with Steady-state Precession (FISP)	Siemens
Balanced Fast Field Echo (FFE)	Phillips
True Steady-State Free Precession (SSFP)	Toshiba

Table 3 MRI based grading of neurovascular compression [8]

Grade	Presentation
I	Mild contact with nerve and vessel
II	Mild distortion/displacement of the nerve root by artery
III	Marked indentation of the nerve root by the vessel

Threapeutic Radiology for Trigeminal Neuralgia

Fluoroscopic Anatomy for Trigeminal Ganglion Neurolysis [14]

The procedural interventions on a patient is carried out in three-dimensional (3D) way based on fluoroscopic images, which are two-dimensional (2D). Hence, it becomes important to view the target in different angles of the fluoroscope so that the actual spatial position of the target aligns with the position of the target in x-ray images. Different views available to the clinician by fluoroscopy are: (a) posteroanterior (PA) view, (b) submental/occipito-mental view, (c) ipsilateral oblique view, and (d) lateral view.

PA view: Intervention of Gasserian ganglion starts with PA view of the face. The patient is placed supine, with the neck slightly extended and the head in neutral position. In PA view, the orbital line and the petrous ridge should be visualized through the orbits (Fig. 6). Besides this, important structures that are visualized are mandible, nasal cavity, maxillary sinus, and supraorbital margin.

Submental view or ipsilateral oblique view: A combination of submental and oblique view is the final view to visualize the foramen ovale (FO), over which the entry point for the cannula or needle in the fluoroscopic image lies. It is also known as the reverse of **occipito-mental (OM) view**. The head is kept extended (usually 45°) and fluoroscope is tilted cranially by 20°–30°. Submental view is considered when *mentonian arch* is clearly visible (Fig. 7). One should be able to identify infraorbital margin, frontal sinus, maxillary sinus, zygomatic arch, coronoid process, and anterior border of ramus of mandible in submental view.

To visualize the FO, the fluoroscope is tilted ipsilateral oblique by approximately 20°, so that the foramen is visualized immediately medial to the anterior border of ramus of mandible, or somewhere between the anterior border (now visualizing as medial border) of ramus of mandible and lateral wall of maxillary sinus. On several

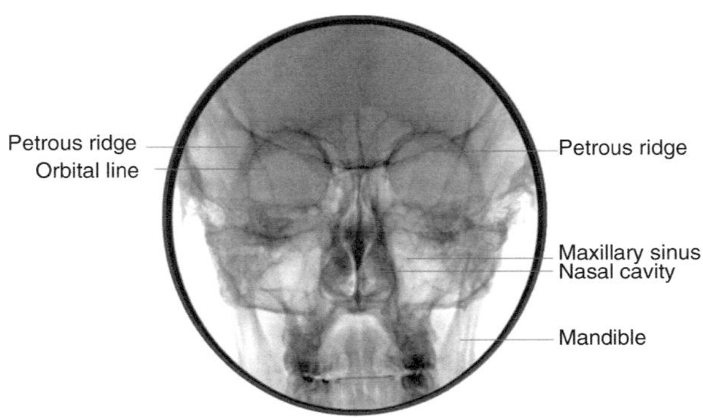

Fig. 6 Anteroposterior view of skull with patient in supine position to decide the side for the percutaneous interventional procedure

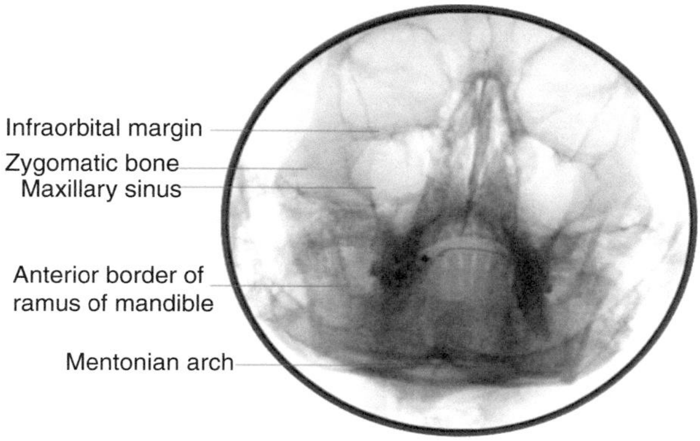

Fig. 7 Submental fluoroscopic view of the skull

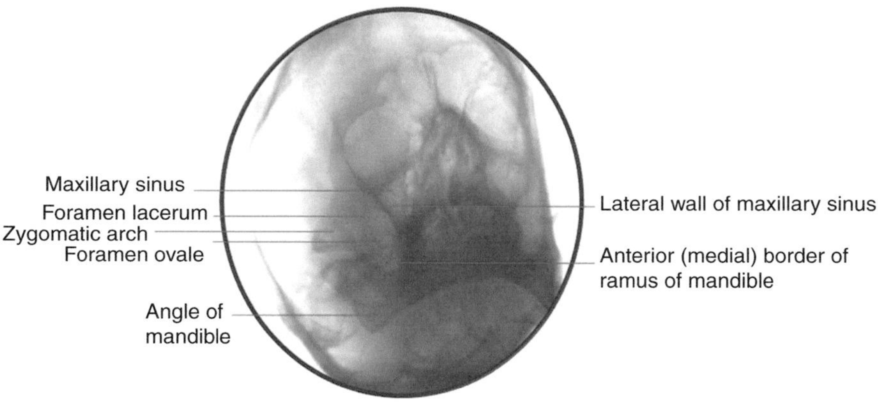

Fig. 8 Anteroposterior fluoroscopic view showing foramen ovale

occasions, one is able to see two different foramen, namely, ovale and spinosum. Usually the FO is bigger in size and obviously, oval in shape (Fig. 8). Needle entry point should be kept on the lateral part of the foramen in the fluoroscopic image, as anatomically, the mandibular nerve is on the lateral part of the FO, and the maxillary and ophthalmic divisions are relatively medial. Needle is inserted in end-on view or tunnel view.

Lateral view: Depth of the needle tip is decided on the lateral view. It is considered appropriate when there is no rotation or tilt of the cranium image seen in relation to the structures on left and right side. Proper superimposition of external auditory meatus, mastoid process and angle/ramus of mandible of left and right side ensure no rotation, and superimposition of orbital floor and mandibular body ensures no tilt. Final position of the needle tip position is confirmed when it is seen in the Meckel's cave, the area inside the cranium close to the apex of petrous part of the temporal bone; the Gasserian ganglion lies there (Fig. 9).

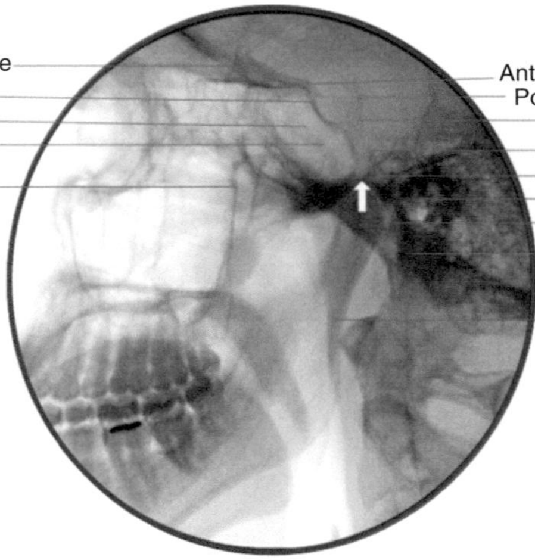

Fig. 9 Lateral fluoroscopic view showing Meckel's cave and the location of Gasserian ganglion

Computed Tomography (CT) Guided Radiofrequency Ablation

Despite disadvantages, computed tomography (CT) remains the only three-dimensional (3D) imaging modality, which can be used in real time for guided procedures. In this procedure, the puncture of Gasserian ganglion is carried out according to Hartel's anterior approach [15]. The best puncture approach to the FO from the skin insertion point is determined by CT scan images. The needle insertion angle and the depth of FO are assessed according to best puncture approach. Repeated CT scan is done to reconfirm the position of needle tip [16]. CT-guided pulsed radiofrequency (RF) thermocoagulation has been found to be safe and effective for classic TGN patients of 70 years or older, including patients with poor-fitness [17]. However, there are contradictory reports when pulsed RF is utilized [18]. CT guided RF ablation has also been tried with success using stereotactic frame; use of stereotactic approach makes it easy to insert the probe into FO [19].

Conclusion

Trigeminal neuralgia is a dreaded disease, which can force the affected person to lead a crippled life. Even though the diagnosis is established mainly based on clinical grounds, radiological tests are important to understand the underlying pathology, and decide on treatment options. MRI is usually the first diagnostic modality. The treating physician needs to be well-versed with the anatomy of the base and lateral view of skull to accurately and safely perform various percutaneous interventional procedures.

References

1. Nicolás S, Andrés S, Osmar T, Inés D, Jorge B, Víctor S. Anatomy of the trigeminal nerve. Key anatomical facts for mri examination of trigeminal neuralgia. Rev Imagenol. 2009;12:28–33.
2. Kontzialis M, Kocak M. Imaging evaluation of trigeminal neuralgia. J Istanb Univ Fac Dent. 2017;51(3 Suppl 1):S62–8.
3. Donia MM, Gamaledin OA, Abdo AM, Desouky SE, Helmy SA. Intracranial neoplastic lesions of the trigeminal nerve: How MRI can help. Egypt J Radiol Nucl Med. 2017;48:1035–41.
4. Majoie CB, Verbeeten B, Dol A, Peeters LM. Trigeminal neuropathy: evaluation with MR imaging. Radiographics. 1995;15:795–811.
5. Tash RR, Sze G, Leslie DR. Trigeminal neuralgia: MR imaging features. Radiology. 1989;172:767–70.
6. Besta R, Shankar YU, Kumar A, Rajasekhar E, Prakash SB. MRI 3D CISS- a novel imaging modality in diagnosing trigeminal neuralgia—a review. J Clin Diagn Res. 2016;10:ZE01–3.
7. Yousry I, Moriggl B, Schmid UD, et al. Trigeminal ganglion and its divisions: detailed anatomic MR imaging with contrast-enhanced 3D constructive interference in the steady state sequences. AJNR Am J Neuroradiol. 2005;26:1128–35.
8. Harsha KJ, Kesavadas C, Chinchure S, Thomas B, Jagtap S. Imaging of vascular causes of trigeminal neuralgia. J Neuroradiol. 2012;39:281–9.
9. Fujiwara S, Sasaki M, Wada T, Kudo K, Hirooka R, Ishigaki D, et al. High-resolution diffusion tensor imaging for the detection of diffusion abnormalities in the trigeminal nerves of patients with trigeminal neuralgia caused by neurovascular compression. J Neuroimaging. 2011;21:e102–8.
10. Jannetta PJ. Arterial compression of the trigeminal nerve at the pons in patients with trigeminal neuralgia. J Neurosurg. 1967;26:159–62.
11. Peker S, Kurtkaya O, Uzün I, Pamir MN. Microanatomy of the central myelin-peripheral myelin transition zone of the trigeminal nerve. Neurosurgery. 2006;59:354–9.
12. Haller S, Etienne L, Kovari E, Varoquaux AD, Urbach H, Becker M. Imaging of neurovascular compression syndrome: trigeminal neuralgia, hemifacial spasm, vestibular paroxysmia, and glossopharyngeal neuralgia. AJNR. 2016;37:1384–92.
13. Hughes MA, Frederickson AM, Branstetter BF, Zho X, Sekula RF. MRI of trigeminal nerve in patients with trigeminal neuralgia secondary to vascular compression. AJR. 2016;206:595–600.
14. Son BC, Kim HS, Kim IS, Yang SH, Lee SW. Percutaneous radiofrequency thermocoagulation under fluoroscopic image-guidance for idiopathic trigeminal neuralgia. J Korean Neurosurg Soc. 2011;50:446–52.
15. Hertel F. Uber die intracranielle injektionsbehandlung der trigeminusneuralgie. Med Klin. 1914;10:582.
16. Lai GH, Tang YZ, Wang XP, Qin HJ, Ni JX. CT-guided percutaneous radiofrequency thermocoagulation for recurrent trigeminal neuralgia after microvascular decompression: a cohort study. Medicine (Baltimore). 2015;94:e1176.
17. Tang YZ, Jin D, Bian JJ, Li XY, Lai GH, Ni JX. Long-term outcome of computed tomography guided percutaneous radiofrequency thermocoagulation for classic trigeminal neuralgia patients older than 70 years. J Craniofac Surg. 2014;25:1292–5.
18. Fang L, Ying S, Tao W, Lan M, Xiaotong Y, Nan J. 3D CT-guided pulsed radiofrequency treatment for trigeminal neuralgia. Pain Pract. 2014;14:16–21.
19. Patil AA, Chamczuk AJ, Nelson B. Stereotactic radiofrequency ablation of trigeminal ganglion with intraoperative CT scans and under general anesthesia. Open J Mod Neurosurg. 2016;6:55–9.
20. Seeburg DP, Northcutt B, Aygun N, Blitz AM. The role of imaging for trigeminal neuralgia: a segmental approach to high-resolution MRI. Neurosurg Clin N Am. 2016;27:315–26.

Pharmacotherapy of Trigeminal Neuralgia

Ayush Agarwal and Manjari Tripathi

Key Points

- Differentiation between classical and symptomatic trigeminal neuralgia (TGN) is important for medical management
- Carbamazepine and Oxcarbazepine are the treatment of choice for TGN
- Add on drugs with variable benefit such as Lamotrigine and Baclofen can be tried
- Combination therapy might be beneficial but no study has compared their efficacy to monotherapy

Introduction

Trigeminal neuralgia (TGN) is a disorder characterized by brief but severe electric shock-like pain, which is abrupt in onset and termination, and is limited to the distribution of one or more divisions of the trigeminal nerve [1]. It is further subclassified into classical (CTN) and symptomatic forms (STN), the latter is associated with a demonstrable lesion on imaging apart from a vascular loop [1]. STN should be suspected when a patient presents with bilateral symptoms or concomitant trigeminal sensory loss. The distinction is important as the treatment for both differs.

A number of treatment options are available for CTN, with the general recommendation being to start with medical therapy, and considering surgical modalities in non-responders [2]. Medical therapy predominantly consists of anti-epileptic drugs (AEDs) such as Carbamazepine and Oxcarbazepine. Fifteen randomized control trials (RCTs) have been done to study the effectiveness of various medications

A. Agarwal · M. Tripathi (✉)
Department of Neurology, All India Institute of Medical Sciences, New Delhi, India

G. P. Rath (ed.), *Handbook of Trigeminal Neuralgia*,
https://doi.org/10.1007/978-981-13-2333-1_8

in TGN, of which eight were placebo-controlled, and in four, Carbamazepine was used as the comparator.

First-Line Pharmacotherapy

Carbamazepine (CBZ) and Oxcarbazepine (OXC) are the first-line treatment for TGN and are prescribed in doses between 200–1200 mg/day and 600–1800 mg/day, respectively. Both of them stabilize the neuronal membranes by inhibiting sodium channels, thereby making them less excitable. They are metabolized by the cytochrome P450 (CYP) system and predominantly excreted in the urine. Both drugs are inducers of the CYP system as well (CBZ>OXC), and therefore, may decrease their own half-lives (auto-induction) as well as others after prolonged administration. The half-life of CBZ decreases from approximately 25 h to 12–17 h after 3 months of treatment. CBZ was found to have robust efficacy in four RCTs [3–6] which had enrolled 147 patients with a number needed to treat (NNT) for attaining important pain relief being 1.7–1.8. It reduced both the intensity and frequency of attacks and was equally effective for both trigger-induced and spontaneous attacks. The exact mechanism of action is unknown and is thought to be related to the blockade of voltage sensitive sodium channels, which results in membrane stabilization and its initial efficacy is approximately 80%, which tends to wane over time due to auto-induction. This effectiveness is hampered by its side effect profile with its number needed to harm (NNH) being 3.4 for minor and 24 for severe adverse events. It is imperative to avoid initial toxicity in the haste of attaining adequate pain relief since patients who experience these avoidable side effects may never again be willing to try one of the most efficacious medications for his pain. Therefore, it is typically started in a low dose and gradually up-titrated. The usual regimen is starting with 100 mg orally twice daily and gradually increasing by 100 mg/day to a maximum dose of 1200 mg/day, with usual maintenance doses between 600 and 800 mg/day. Common ones include drowsiness, nausea, vertigo, ataxia, dizziness, diplopia, hyponatremia, and derangement of liver functions. These are usually dose dependent and resolve over a few days. Severe ones are myelo-suppression including aplastic anemia, allergic rash and Stevens-Johnson syndrome (SJS) and lymphadenopathy. The incidence of SJS and toxic epidermal necrolysis are especially high in HLA-B1502 harbouring individuals, and therefore, screening for the same should be done, whenever possible. Complete blood counts, serum sodium and liver function tests should therefore, be routinely monitored. Serum CBZ levels should be monitored 2–3 weeks after starting treatment and once in 3 months thereafter to ensure therapeutic drug levels. Between 6% and 10% patients are unable to tolerate CBZ altogether. Women of childbearing age, using oral contraceptives, should be intimated about the increased chances of contraceptive failure with CBZ and to be informed about switching to other modalities if possible.

Oxcarbazepine (OXC) has similar efficacy to CBZ which was documented in three RCTs with the latter as the comparator. It is preferred because of its better tolerability and decreased drug interactions as compared to CBZ [7]. It is a pro-drug that is rapidly converted to its active metabolite. This is a weak enzyme inducer and therefore has lesser drug interactions. It is usually started at a dose of 150 mg twice daily, and the dose increased by 300 mg every 3 days to a maximum dose of 1800 mg. The usual effective dose is 300–600 mg twice daily.

Second-Line Pharmacotherapy

The second-line of treatment is based on sparse evidence and includes add-on to lamotrigine or a switch therapy with lamotrigine, baclofen, or pimozide, the later drug is seldom in clinical practice owing to possible complications of extrapyramidal symptoms.

Lamotrigine is thought to act in a similar manner to CBZ/OXC and has been shown to be superior to placebo in TGN patients' refractory to CBZ [8]. It is initiated at a low dose of 25 mg/day, and very gradually up-titrated to its target dose of 200–400 mg/day. The side effects include dizziness, nausea, ataxia and blurred vision. Rash develops in 7–10% cases during the initial therapy and gradually resolves with continued treatment. However, therapy with lamotrigine should be discontinued in cases of SJS or lymphadenopathy. The slower the titration of the drug, the more unlikely is the occurrence of these side effects.

Baclofen, a skeletal muscule relaxant, suppresses excitatory neurotransmission by acting as a gamma aminobutyric acid ($GABA_B$) receptor agonist. It has been shown to have 70% efficacy at doses between 10 and 60 mg/day, in double-blinded trials [9]. However, follow up studies over the next 5 years suggested that persistent benefit was present only in 30% cases with 17% having a recurrence within the first 6 months of treatment and 22% having refractory symptoms by 1.5 years. It is usually initiated in doses of 5–10 mg thrice daily and doses increased by 10 mg on alternate days to a maximum dose of 90 mg. The typical effective dose is 50–60 mg/day in divided doses. It is renally excreted, and therefore can be given in patients with liver ailments, unlike most other medications used in TGN. The discontinuation should be gradual to avoid potential side effects of confusion, seizures, and hallucinations. The commonly encountered side effects include somnolence, lassitude, dizziness, and gastrointestinal discomfort. Routine blood tests are not required for patients taking baclofen. It also shows synergistic actions with CBZ and therefore patients showing inadequate symptomatic benefit can be tried on a combination of the two drugs. However, an RCT demonstrating such efficacy is presently lacking.

Alternative Pharmacotherapy

Many other AEDs have been studied in case control or open label studies and have shown modest benefit. There is insufficient evidence to advocate or refute the effectiveness of all of them. These drugs include phenytoin, clonazepam, gabapentin, pregabalin, levetiracetam, topiramate, tocainide, and valproate. Considering the diversity in the mechanism of action, combination therapy might be beneficial but no study till date has compared monotherapy with polytherapy.

Phenytoin was the first drug ever to be used, with promising results, but no RCT has been published on the same till date [10]. It is believed to bring about pain relief in approximately 60% patients. However, due to tachyphylaxis, this effect is short-lived and sustained benefit is seen only in 25% patients. Its most important practical value lies in the fact that it can be used in patients presenting with acute neuralgic crisis. Unlike other AEDs, it can be given intravenously with a loading dose of 12 mg/kg, at an infusion rate of 50 mg/min for quick cessation of an acute attack.

Gabapentin showed moderate efficacy when used alone or in combination with CBZ/OXC. It is usually initiated at a dosage of 300 mg/day, increased by 300 mg/ every 2–3 days for a maximum dose of 3600 mg, prescribed in divided doses. Its advantage is relative absence of significant drug interactions. Minor side effects like drowsiness, dizziness, confusion, nausea, and ankle swelling may occur which are self-limiting [11].

Pregabalin, a structural analogue of gabapentin, prescribed in doses of 150–600 mg/day, also showed efficacy similar to gabapentin, with better results in patients having concomitant chronic facial pain. More than 50% reduction in pain was witnessed in approximately 74% TGN patients, with only minor efficacy reduction over the next one year [12]. Ataxia and tremor may occur as side-effects of pregabalin.

Topiramate is effective when given at a dose of 100–400 mg/day. In a study of eight patients it was found to be effective in 75% of them [13]. The side effects include sedation, dizziness, cognitive impairment, blurred vision, fatigue, and weight loss.

Levetiracetam was studied for efficacy in a pilot study with 10 patients, with doses upto 4000 mg/day and more than 50% symptomatic improvement was reported in 40% cases [14]. Adverse reactions may occur in the form of drowsiness, nasopharyngitis, and influenza on initiation of the drug.

Tizanidine, a centrally acting alpha adrenergic agonist, was studied in ten patients with double-blind crossover design. Out of these patients eight showed some improvement in symptomatology. However, all patients had symptom recurrence when followed up at 3 months interval.

Valproate, an anticonvulsant drug with GABAergic properties has been used with mixed results in patients with TGN in doses between 600 and 1600 mg/day. Desai et al. [15] reported symptomatic benefit in patients who responded poorly to CBZ, with 8 out of 10 patients reporting more than 50% symptomatic benefit. It is usually started at a dose of 250 mg thrice a day, and gradually up-titrated according to efficacy and side effect profile. Gastrointestinal side effects like dyspepsia can occur and be prevented by using the enteric coated formulation. It is teratogenic and can cause polycystic ovarian disease, hence, avoided in young females. Weight gain and liver function abnormalities are other side effects and therefore, liver function tests should be done before starting therapy.

Tricyclic antidepressants, although effective in neuropathic pain, have no evidence of efficacy in TGN. A single study found Clomipramine to be superior to Amitriptyline for the treatment of TGN, probably reflecting better 5-HT blockade [16].

No placebo controlled studies have been conducted for STN till date. Most published literature is small open-label studies dealing with TGN in multiple sclerosis. Lamotrigine, gabapentin, and topiramate have all been shown to be effective, alone or in combination with CBZ. **Misoprostol**, a prostaglandin E1 analogue, showed efficacy in a study that enrolled 25 patients. However, there is insufficient evidence to support or refute the efficacy of any of these drugs for the management of STN.

American Academy of Neurology (AAN) and European Federation of Neurological Society (EFNS) guidelines [17] recommend the use of CBZ/OXC as the first line of treatment for TGN, with early referral for surgical management if these drugs are ineffective (Table 1). If surgery is unlikely, due to whatever reason, there is insufficient data to recommend the next line of management. However, add on/switch treatment with lamotrigine or baclofen seems to be the best available option. The efficacy of other drugs is uncertain and can be tried as deemed necessary. Treatment should be individualized and titrated according to treatment effect and drugs that cease to be effective can be re-introduced after a period of several months, with subsequent benefit [18].

Table 1 American Association of Neurology (AAN/European Federation of Neurological Society (EFNS) Guidelines [14]

Which drugs effectively treat Classic Trigeminal Neuralgia (CTN) pain?	
Strong evidence	Strong evidence supports that carbamazepine should be offered to treat CTN pain **(Level A)**
Good evidence	Good evidence supports that oxcarbazepine should be considered to treat CTN pain **(Level B)**
Clinical context	The two drugs to consider as first-line therapy in TGN are CBZ (200–1200 mg/day) and OXC (600–1800 mg/day). Although the evidence for CBZ is stronger than for OXC, the latter may pose fewer safety concerns
Weak evidence	Weak evidence supports that baclofen, lamotrigine, and pimozide may be considered to treat CTN pain **(Level C)**
Good evidence	Good evidence supports that topical ophthalmic anesthesia should not be considered to treat CTN pain **(Level B)**
Clinical context	There is little evidence to guide the clinician on the treatment of TGN patients who fail first-line therapy. Some evidence supports add-on therapy with lamotrigine or a switch to baclofen
Which drugs effectively treat Symptomatic Trigeminal Neuralgia (STN) pain?	
Insufficient evidence	There is insufficient evidence to support or refute the effectiveness of any medication in treating pain in STN **(Level U)**
Clinical context	The effect of other drugs commonly used in neuropathic pain is unknown There are no published studies directly comparing polytherapy with monotherapy
Is there evidence of efficacy of intravenous administration of drugs in acute exacerbations of TGN?	
Insufficient evidence	There is insufficient evidence to support or refute the efficacy of intravenous medications for the treatment of pain from TGN **(Level U)**

TGN Trigeminal neuralgia

Conclusion

Although various AEDs are available for the management of TGN, carbamazepine remain the gold-standard for the initial management. Add-on or switch therapy with second-line drugs may be tried in patients who are not the candidates for surgery. Various alternative medications of guarded efficacy may be tried as monotherapy or polytherapy based on the response to alleviation of symptoms. In medically refractory cases surgical options may be explored.

References

1. International Headache Society. The international classification of headache disorders: 2nd Edition. Cephalalgia. 2004;24(Suppl 1):9–160.
2. Obermann M. Treatment options in trigeminal neuralgia. Ther Adv Neurol Disord. 2010;3:107–15.
3. Campbell FG, Graham JG, Zilkha KJ. Clinical trial of carbamazepine (tegretol) in trigeminal neuralgia. J Neurol Neurosurg Psychiatry. 1966;29:265–7.
4. Killian JM, Fromm GH. Carbamazepine in the treatment of neuralgia. Arch Neurol. 1968;19:129–36.
5. Nicol CF. A four year double blind study of tegretol in facial pain. Headache. 1969;9:54–7.
6. Rockcliff BW, Davis EH. Controlled sequential trials of carbamazepine in trigeminal neuralgia. Arch Neurol. 1996;15:129–36.
7. Kutluay E, McCague K, D'Souza J, Beydoun A. Safety and tolerability of oxcarbazepine in elderly patients with epilepsy. Epilepsy Behav. 2003;4:175–80.
8. Zakrzewska JM, Chaudhry Z, Nurmikko TJ, Patton DW, Mullens EL. Lamotrigine (Lamictal) in refractory trigeminal neuralgia: results from a double-blind placebo controlled crossover trial. Pain. 1997;73:223–30.
9. Fromm GH, Terrence CF, Chattha AS. Baclofen in the treatment of trigeminal neuralgia: double-blind study and long-term follow-up. Ann Neurol. 1984;15:240–4.
10. Sindrup SH, Jensen TS. Pharmacotherapy of trigeminal neuralgia. Clin J Pain. 2002;18:22–7.
11. Lemos L, Flores S, Oliveira P, Almeida A. Gabapentin supplemented with ropivacain block of trigger points improves pain control and quality of life in trigeminal neuralgia patients when compared with gabapentin alone. Clin J Pain. 2008;24:64–75.
12. Obermann M, Yoon MS, Sensen K, Maschke M, Diener HC, Katsarava Z. Efficacy of pregabalin in the treatment of trigeminal neuralgia. Cephalalgia. 2008;28:174–81.
13. Domingues RB, Kuster GW, Aquino CC. Treatment of trigeminal neuralgia with low doses of topiramate. Arq Neuropsiquiatr. 2007;65:792–4.
14. Jorns TP, Johnston A, Zakrzewska JM. Pilot study to evaluate the efficacy and tolerability of levetiracetam in treatment of patients with trigeminal neuralgia. Eur J Neurol. 2009;16:740–4.
15. Desai N, Shah K, Gandhi I. Baclofen sodium valproate combination in carbamazepine resistant trigeminal neuralgia: a double blind clinical trial. Cephalalgia. 1991;II(Suppl):321–2.
16. Carasso RL, Yehuda S, Streifler M. Clomipramine and amitriptyline in the treatment of severe pain. Int J Neurosci. 1979;9:191–4.
17. Cruccu G, Gronseth G, Alksne J, Argoff C, Brainin M, Burchiel K, Nurmikko T, Zakrzewska JM, American Academy of Neurology Society, European Federation of Neurological Society. AAN-EFNS guidelines on trigeminal neuralgia management. Eur J Neurol. 2008;15:1013–28.
18. William P. Cheshire. Trigeminal neuralgia: a guide to drug choice. CNS Drugs. 1997;7:98–110.

Part II

Peripheral Nerve Blocks for Trigeminal Neuralgia

Medications for Interventional Pain Management in Trigeminal Neuralgia

Siddharth Chavali

Key Points

- The pharmacological agents most commonly used in the management of trigeminal neuralgia include local anesthetics, corticosteroids, and neurolytic agents
- Although of historical importance, neurolytic agents are now losing ground to newer modalities of treatment, in part due to their unfavourable side effect profile

Introduction

Clinicians have been searching for means to alleviate incapacitating pain for a long time. Perineural injection of various substances found to reduce pain, by interrupting neural conduction, chemical neurolysis, or other mechanisms of action. The medications most commonly administered during interventional procedures for pain management include local anesthetics, corticosteroids, and neurolytic agents. This chapter contains a brief review of the most commonly used agents in interventional procedures for trigeminal neuralgia (TGN).

S. Chavali (✉)
Department of Neuroanaesthesiology and Critical Care, All India Institute of Medical Sciences (AIIMS), New Delhi, India

G. P. Rath (ed.), *Handbook of Trigeminal Neuralgia*,
https://doi.org/10.1007/978-981-13-2333-1_9

Local Anesthetics

Local anesthetics (LA) act on any nerve fiber to interrupt conduction in a reversible manner, without damaging the neural tract. This reversible blockade makes these agents suited to both diagnostic as well as therapeutic procedures. All local anesthetic agents have similar structures with an aromatic benzene ring and an amino group joined by a linkage. These agents are classified into two groups based on the nature of this linkage, which determines their metabolism. Amino-ester LA are broken down rapidly by plasma cholinesterase to a common metabolite, para-amino benzoate (PABA), which is excreted in the urine. PABA is a known allergen, but rapid metabolism of these drugs renders them relatively less toxic. Amino-amide LA are metabolized in the liver by the cytochrome P450 system. This class is less allergenic, and more commonly utilized in the clinical setting.

Mechanism of Action

LAs act by reversibly inhibiting neural impulse conduction. The LA molecules traverse the neural membranes to block sodium channels, and inhibit sodium influx; hence, the drug needs to be injected in close proximity to the nerve. Only a 5–10 mm segment of the nerve needs to be blocked to inhibit neural firing. The ability of a LA to effectively block neuronal conduction depends on the following factors:

pH: influences the *speed of onset* of the block. The ability of a LA to diffuse through membrane and block sodium channels depends on the ability of these molecules to dissociate at physiological pH. In general, the lower the pKa that the LA has, the faster the onset of action. The addition of bicarbonate to LAs hastens their onset, by raising the pH, and hence the amount of non-ionized LA for diffusion across the neuronal membrane. Also, CO_2 diffuses across the axonal membrane and lowers intracellular pH, increasing the ionized fraction of the LA available to block sodium channels.

In addition to this, *duration of action* of the LA may be affected by the **volume** and **concentration** of the injectate, the presence or absence of **vasoconstrictor** additives, **site** of injection, and the **temperature** of the solution. The addition of agents like epinephrine and phenylephrine reverse the intrinsic vasodilation caused by LAs and reduce their systemic absorption, increasing the amount of LA available to block the nerve over a period of time. Injection of these agents into highly vascular sites such as the caudal epidural space tend to result in shorter durations of action due to systemic uptake.

Individual Agents

Lidocaine

This is the most widely used local anesthetic agent. It has a short onset of action (0.5–5 min) and a short duration of action (0.5–3 h). The therapeutic index is also wider, compared to other LAs. Typical preparations for clinical use range between

0.5% and 2%, although final concentration is often diluted by adding a corticosteroid. The maximal safe dose is about 3 mg/kg, which increases to 7 mg/kg with the addition of epinephrine.

Bupivacaine

It has a longer duration of action than lidocaine (2–5 h), but onset of action is also slower (5–20 min). Bupivacaine is usually used in concentrations of 0.125–0.75% without epinephrine. Bupivacaine has a more cardiotoxic profile as compared to lidocaine, especially if injected intravenously.

Ropivacaine

Is structurally related to bupivacaine, but is a pure S(−) enantiomer, as compared to a racemate [1]. It was developed for the purpose of reducing potential toxicity and improving sensorimotor block. Concentrations range from 0.2% to 1%, and cardiotoxicity is significantly lower than bupivacaine, making it more suited for large-volume blocks. Recent studies have shown that peripheral analgesic block with ropivacaine with ongoing therapy led to a significant dose reduction in oral therapy, as well as improved pain scores on follow-up [2].

Adverse Effects

LAs may lead to local as well as systemic toxicity. Local toxicity may be seen with highly concentrated solutions, or intraneural injection may lead to neurotoxicity even at normal drug dosages. Systemic toxicity occurs in about 7–20/10,000 peripheral nerve blocks [3, 4]. Toxicity is usually associated with excessive drug, intravascular injection, or impaired metabolism or elimination. CNS symptoms consist of metallic taste, perioral numbness, and generalized seizure activity. Cardiovascular effects include arrhythmias, hypotension due to vasodilation, decreased inotropy, and cardiac collapse. Potent lipophilic agents are more cardiotoxic, and resuscitation may be both difficult and prolonged [5]. Intralipid 20% has been proven effective in the treatment of bupivacaine induced cardiotoxicity, via the extraction of lipophilic LAs, with a bolus of 1–2 mL/kg followed by an infusion of 0.25–0.5mL/kg [6].

Allergic reactions to LA are uncommon, and the majority are caused by PABA, which is an end product of amino-ester LA metabolism. Amino-amide LA are not associated with any significant allergic potential. Paraben preservatives are structurally similar to PABA, and may manifest as a delayed allergic reaction with minor, self-limited cutaneous rashes. Bisulfite preservatives may trigger reactivity in patients with known food allergies or sulfa allergies, and this should be borne in mind.

Corticosteroids

These are commonly used drugs in pain practice due to their potent anti-inflammatory properties. All corticosteroids have both glucocorticoid as well as mineralocorticoid activity. Agents with significant glucocorticoid action and minimal mineralocorticoid action such as dexamethasone, methylprednisolone and triamcinolone are preferred for peripheral nerve blockade.

Mechanism of Action

The primary mechanism of action seems to be their ability to inhibit prostaglandin synthesis, resulting in reduced inflammation, as well as by reducing cytokine release by immune cells [7]. The anti-inflammatory effects of corticosteroids are also seen at the vascular level. They block transfer of immune mediators across vascular basement membrane, reduce superoxide radical release and also decrease capillary permeability, resulting in reduced tissue edema. Steroid receptors are present in the central as well as peripheral nervous systems and may be involved in neuronal growth and plasticity [7]. Corticosteroids have also been proven to reduce spontaneous firing in injured nerves, which may lead to decreased neuropathic pain [8].

Methylprednisolone

Methylprednisolone acetate has a slightly lower glucocorticoid potency as compared to betamethasone but similar anti-inflammatory action to prednisolone, with an intermediate duration of action. It is approved for intraarticular and soft tissue injections for osteoarthritis, bursitis, tenosynovitis and rheumatoid arthritis [9]. Polyethelene glycol is used as a suspending agent in methylprednisolone acetate, which has been reported to cause arachnoiditis with accidental intrathecal injections [10].

Triamcinolone

It is available in three preparations: diacetate, hexacetonide and acetonide salts. Duration of action is least with diacetate, and greatest with the acetonide salts. Triamcinolone has similar glucocorticoid activity to methylprednisolone with a long half-life. It is however associated with a greater incidence of adverse effects including fat atrophy and hypopigmentation.

Dexamethasone

Dexamethasone is a potent synthetic glucocorticoid and has been used widely for the treatment of postoperative nausea and to improve recovery following major surgical procedures. A few studies have proven the efficacy of this drug in prolonging the analgesic duration of peripheral neural blockade. A study by Han et al suggested that early administration of dexamethasone produced significant anti-nociceptive activity in trigeminal neuropathic pain [11].

Adverse Effects

Injections of corticosteroids should be avoided if possible in high-risk patients such as patients with ulcerative colitis, poorly controlled hypotension, congestive cardiac failure, or a history of allergies. Adverse effects of injected steroids include a transient increase in pain for up to 48 h hours in 10% of patients.

- Intraarticular injection may lead to osteonecrosis, infection, or tendon rupture
- Intraspinal injections may be associated with arachnoiditis, meningitis and conus medullaris syndrome
- Diabetic patients may become hyperglycemic after administration of steroids
- Frequent, high-dose injections may lead to adrenal cortical insufficiency
- Slow release formulations of glucocorticoids have been associated with a delayed allergic response [12]
- Other side effects include hypopigmentation, flushing, subcutaneous fat atrophy, peripheral edema, etc.
- Repeated dosing may result in Cushingoid changes

Neurolytic Agents

Neurolysis is defined as the selective, iatrogenic destruction of neural tissue to secure pain relief. The use of neurolytic agents has long been studied in the treatment of pain. The first reported use of neurolysis in trigeminal neuralgia was done by Schloesser in 1904, who used alcohol [13]. These agents are nonspecific in destroying all nerve fiber types and their spread cannot be controlled, making their use controversial in the treatment of non-malignant pain.

Mechanism of Action

Chemical neurolytic agents such as phenol, alcohol and glycerol cause a dose-dependent, nonselective denaturing of proteins leading to necrosis, Wallerian degeneration, and a complete conduction block in all the fibers contained in the nerve bundle (Table 1).

Alcohol

The use of alcohol as a neurolytic agent has reduced due to its diffusibility and solubility. 100% alcohol is commonly used, and a recent study has reported its long-term effectiveness in treatment of trigeminal neuralgia [14]. Alcohol leads to

Table 1 Neurolytic agents used for the interventional management of trigeminal neuralgia

Agent	Concentration (%)	Adverse properties	Toxicity
Alcohol	50–100	Painful, increased risk of neuritis	Disulfiram like reaction
Phenol	3–12	Duration of action, affinity for vasculature	CNS and CVS manifestations
Glycerol	50	Diffusion	Severe headache, local dysesthesia

nonselective neuronal destruction by extracting cholesterol and phospholipids as well as by precipitating lipoproteins [15]. Its use with peripheral nerves has declined because of the marked pain it causes on injection and its tendency to produce neuritis. Preceding the alcohol injection with a local anesthetic diminishes the pain of injection but may lessen the neurolytic effect because of dilution.

Phenol

The nonselective neural destruction caused by phenol is similar to that of alcohol. It can be used in concentrations ranging from 3% to 12%, and it can be injected epidurally or peripherally. Unlike alcohol, phenol is not painful on injection, and diffuses poorly, especially when mixed with glycerine [16]. Phenol has local anesthetic properties, and on successful placement, pain is relieved immediately. This block fades in intensity over the first 24 h, leaving a neurolytic effect of lesser intensity.

Glycerol

Häkanson first reported a success rate of 86% in the treatment of facial pain using glycerol [17]; since then, it has become popular for this indication. When used in a concentration of 50%, it causes selective destruction of nerve fibers, with facial sensation usually remaining intact. Axonolysis, myelin swelling, and lipid droplets in the cytoplasm have been described, with ongoing nerve damage that continues for weeks. It is extremely viscous and difficult to inject through fine needles. When injection along peripheral nerves is performed, aliquots of 0.1 mL are recommended.

Adverse Effects

- ***Skin necrosis***: This is due to damage of the vascular supply to the skin, causing ischemia. Necrosis of muscles, blood vessels, and other soft tissues has also been reported.
- ***Neuritis***: The reported incidence of neuritis is up to 10 percent. It is caused by partial destruction of somatic nerve and subsequent regeneration. Neuritis occurs when the nerve cell body is not destroyed and manifests as hyperesthesia/dysesthesia that may be worse than the original pain, and is one of the limiting factors in the use of chemical neurolysis.
- ***Anesthesia Dolorosa***: This is a poorly understood condition where the patient complains of numbness caused by long-term loss of afferent input and the resultant CNS changes. Management of this problem is pharmacotherapy with the use of tricyclic antidepressants and anticonvulsants.
- ***Prolonged motor paralysis***: It occurs rarely and is usually self-limiting.
- ***Systemic complications***: These include hypotension secondary to sympathetic block and systemic toxic reactions, arrhythmias, hypotension, and CNS excitation or depression.

Conclusion

Several drugs have been evaluated for their usefulness in the treatment of TGN, however, no single mode of therapy has proven to be superior to others. As newer advances such as radiofrequency lesioning and prolotherapy come to the fore, the utility of perineural injection of various agents may need to be reconsidered.

References

1. Hansen TG. Ropivacaine: a pharmacological review. Expert Rev Neurother. 2004;4:781–91.
2. Lemos L, Fontes R, Flores S, Oliveira P, Almeida A. Effectiveness of the association between carbamazepine and peripheral analgesic block with ropivacaine for the treatment of trigeminal neuralgia. J Pain Res. 2010;3:201–12.
3. Mulroy MF. Systemic toxicity and cardiotoxicity from local anesthetics: incidence and preventive measures. Reg Anesth Pain Med. 2002;27:556–61.
4. Corman SL, Skledar SJ. Use of lipid emulsion to reverse local anesthetic-induced toxicity. Ann Pharmacother. 2007;41:1873–7.
5. Zink W, Graf BM. The toxicity of local anesthetics: the place of ropivacaine and levobupivacaine. Curr Opin Anaesthesiol. 2008;21:645–50.
6. Zausig YA, Zink W, Keil M, et al. Lipid emulsion improves recovery from bupivacaine-induced cardiac arrest, but not from ropivacaine- or mepivacaine-induced cardiac arrest. Anesth Analg. 2009;109:1323–6.
7. Mensah-Nyagan AG, Meyer L, Schaeffer V, Kibaly C, Patte-Mensah C. Evidence for a key role of steroids in the modulation of pain. Psychoneuroendocrinology. 2009;34(Suppl 1):S169–77.
8. Watanabe S, Bruera E. Corticosteroids as adjuvant analgesics. J Pain Symptom Manage. 1994;9:442–5.
9. Pelletier JP, Mineau F, Raynauld JP, Woessner JF, Gunja-Smith Z, Martel-Pelletier J. Intraarticular injections with methylprednisolone acetate reduce osteoarthritic lesions in parallel with chondrocyte stromelysin synthesis in experimental osteoarthritis. Arthritis Rheum. 1994;37:414–23.
10. Johnson A, Ryan MD, Roche J. Depo-Medrol and myelographic arachnoiditis. Med J Aust. 1991;155:18–20.
11. Han SR, Yeo SP, Lee MK, Bae YC, Ahn DK. Early dexamethasone relieves trigeminal neuropathic pain. J Dent Res. 2010;89:915–20.
12. Laberge L, Pratt M. Immediate and delayed hypersensitivity to systemic corticosteroids: 2 case reports. Dermat Contact Atopic Occup Drug. 2012;23:288–90.
13. Harris W. An analysis of 1,433 cases of paroxysmal trigeminal neuralgia (trigeminal-tic) and the end-results of gasserian alcohol injection. Brain. 1940;63:209–24.
14. Han KR, Chae YJ, Lee JD, Kim C. Trigeminal nerve block with alcohol for medically intractable classic trigeminal neuralgia: long-term clinical effectiveness on pain. Int J Med Sci. 2017;14:29–36.
15. Han KR, Kim C. Brief report: the long-term outcome of mandibular nerve block with alcohol for the treatment of trigeminal neuralgia. Anesth Analg. 2010;111:550–3.
16. Jefferson A. Trigeminal root and ganglion injections using phenol in glycerine for the relief of trigeminal neuralgia. J Neurol Neurosurg Psychiatry. 1963;26:345–52.
17. Håkanson S. Trigeminal neuralgia treated by the injection of glycerol into the trigeminal cistern. Neurosurgery. 1981;9:638–46.

Supraorbital Nerve Block

Siddharth Chavali and Girija Prasad Rath

Key Points

- Supraorbital neuralgia is a rare disorder with pain limited to the distribution of supraorbital nerve
- It may be triggered by compression of the nerve along its course
- Owing to the vascularity of the forehead, care should be taken during nerve block to avoid intravascular injection of drugs

Introduction

Supraorbital neuralgia is an uncommon pain syndrome which may present with a typical history of shock-like pain restricted to the area just above the eyebrow. It is also known as **Goggle headache** [1] **or Swimmer's headache** [2]**.** It is associated with a characteristic triad of symptoms, namely: (1) Pain limited to the area innervated by the supraorbital nerve; (2) Tenderness on supraorbital notch or area distributed by the nerve; and (3) Symptomatic relief following nerve blockade. The pain presents with an intermittent or chronic pattern. The pain presents with an intermittent or chronic pattern with periods of varied severity. The hallmark of supraorbital neuralgia is localized pain in or above the eyebrow (sometimes extending into the scalp region) [3]. There may be symptoms of altered sensation and typical features of neuralgia, such as pain triggered by relatively innocuous mechanisms.

S. Chavali · G. P. Rath (✉)
Department of Neuroanaesthesiology and Critical Care Neurosciences Centre,
All India Institute of Medical Sciences, New Delhi, India

G. P. Rath (ed.), *Handbook of Trigeminal Neuralgia*,
https://doi.org/10.1007/978-981-13-2333-1_10

Etiopathogenesis of Supraorbital Neuralgia

Although the exact etiopathogenesis remains unclear, supraorbital neuralgia may occur due to nerve entrapment at the point of its exit from the skull after any facial trauma [4, 5]. It may be a sequel to facial reconstruction surgery involving the eyebrow and eyelids; the resultant pain may not present for several years until significant expansion of scar tissue causes entrapment of the nerve [6]. This neuralgia may also be caused by ill-fitting eyewear, and subsequently, presents as pain in the middle of the forehead, that resolves spontaneously upon removal of the glasses. It is typically described as a steadily increasing headache with maximal pain at the point where the nerve is being compressed. This phenomenon may be misdiagnosed as frontal sinusitis. Supraorbital nerve entrapment may also present as unilateral or bilateral headaches, often presenting just prior to menses, or may be triggered by bright lights causing the patient to squint.

Anatomy

The face receives sensory innervation via the trigeminal nerve (V), which subsequently divides to form the ophthalmic (V1), maxillary (V2), and mandibular (V3) nerves, innervating discrete areas of the face. The ophthalmic division innervates the areas of the scalp, nose, forehead, conjunctiva, and cornea. Within the orbit, the ophthalmic nerve forms the frontal nerve, which then divides into the supraorbital and supratrochlear nerves. The supraorbital nerve exits the skull via the supraorbital foramen with the supraorbital artery, then courses upward squeezed in between the elevator palpebrae muscle and the periosteum of the skull. It then branches into medial and lateral branches; the medial branch provides innervation to the skin of the scalp upto the lambdoidal suture, while the lateral branch courses superiorly and laterally, innervating the upper eyelid and forehead. Both branches of the nerve are often extensively entwined with arteries.

Indications

- Pain relief for trigeminal neuralgia in ophthalmic division
- Pain due to acute herpes zoster in ophthalmic division
- Pain due to isolated supraorbital neuralgia

Contraindications

- Allergy or sensitivity to anesthetic agents
- Infection at the injection site
- Distortion of anatomical landmarks
- Uncooperative patient

Techniques

Landmark Guided Technique (Classical Approach)

- The supraorbital nerve courses through the supraorbital foramen, which is located 2–3 cm lateral to the midline, at the lower margin of the supraorbital ridge (Fig. 1).
- The foramen can usually be palpated along the mid-pupillary line. The patient is asked to look straight and the physician draws an imaginary vertical line drawn through the pupil toward the supraorbital ridge. On palpation along the ridge a notch is felt which is the supraorbital foramen.
- A 25-gauge needle is introduced perpendicularly to the skin, just above the supraorbital notch.
- Care should be taken not to penetrate the foramen, and 1.5–2 mL of local anesthetic solution can be injected after negative aspiration.
- If the patient reports paresthesia during injection, the needle is withdrawn 1–2 mm to avoid accidental intraneural injection.
- Placement of a roll of gauze under the orbital rim immediately after injection of the local anesthetic agent helps prevent swelling of the upper eyelid by spread of the solution through the loose alveolar tissue.

Ultrasound Guided Technique

- The patient is asked to lie supine. The supraorbital notch on the affected side may be identified by palpation. The skin over the notch is prepared with antiseptic solution.
- A high frequency linear ultrasound transducer is placed in the transverse position over the supraorbital foramen which visualized as an interruption in the continuity of the hyper-echoic supraorbital ridge (Fig. 2).

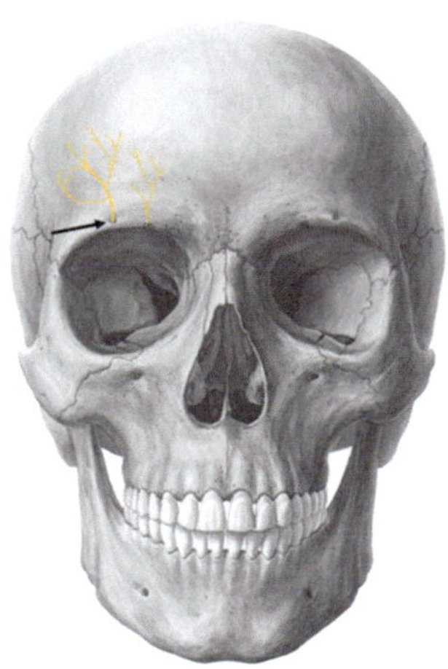

Fig. 1 Supraorbital nerve coming out of supraorbital foramen (site for the nerve block)

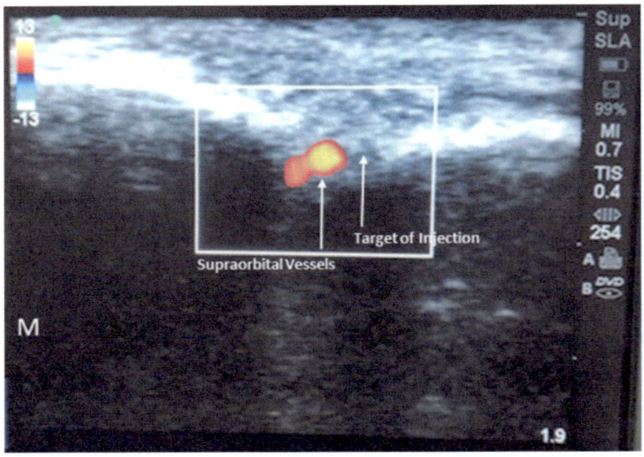

Fig. 2 Ultrasound guided supraorbital nerve block

- Colour Doppler may be used to identify the exiting supraorbital artery, which accompanies the supraorbital nerve upto this point.
- A 25-gauge needle is advanced using an out-of-plane approach until the needle tip lies close to the nerve. Care should be taken to ensure that the needle does not enter the supraorbital foramen.

Drugs

- Commonly used local anesthetic agents are lidocaine 1% or bupivacaine 0.25–0.5%.
- Lidocaine has a faster onset of action (3–5 min) and a duration of action of approximately 30–60 min.
- Bupivacaine has a slower onset of action (5 min) and a duration of action of approximately 4–5 h.
- Adding sodium bicarbonate to the local anesthetic solution may reduce pain associated with injection and also shorten the onset of action.
- Addition of epinephrine (1:200,000) may lead to an increase in the duration of the block.
- Use of adjunct steroids such as triamcinolone or methylprednisolone may provide longer duration of analgesia.
- Chemical neurolysis may be attempted with alcohol or phenol.
- Botulinum toxin has been shown to be of benefit, probably due to muscular entrapment of the nerve. Risks include blepharoptosis and paraesthesia, and pain relief is usually transient.

Complications and Management

- The forehead and scalp have rich vascular supply. Hence, the total dose of local anaesthetic should be carefully calculated for safe administration. In the event of hematoma formation, direct pressure should be applied at the injection site for 5–15 min. Increased vascularity of tissue also increases the risk of hematoma or ecchymosis formation. Administration of cold packs after the block reduces the incidence of post-procedure pain and bleeding.
- Infection may rarely spread along the venous drainage of the superior ophthalmic vein to the cavernous sinus with intracranial extension.
- There are possibilities of failure to anesthetize, nerve damage, and swelling in the eyelid.
- Repeated injections of steroids may cause localized lipodystrophy and skin indentation, which may be avoided by use of fan technique during injection.

Outcomes

There are no randomized controlled trials showing sustained benefit from supraorbital nerve block/lesioning. However, the nerve block in patients with refractory migraine located to the forehead may have reported lasting (>6 months) benefit. Similarly, surgical release and peripheral nerve stimulation can sometimes be effective in patients with refractory neuralgia.

References

1. Pestronk A, Pestronk S. Goggle migraine. New Engl J Med. 1983;308:226–7.
2. Indo T, Takahashi A. Swimmer's migraine. Headache. 1990;30:485–7.
3. Headache Classification Committee of the International Headache Society (IHS). The International Classification of Headache Disorders, 3rd edition (beta version). Cephalalgia Int J Headache. 2013;33:629–808.
4. Caminero A, Pareja J. Supraorbital neuralgia: a clinical study. Cephalalgia. 2001;21:216–23.
5. Sjaastad O, Petersen HC, Bakketeig LS. Supraorbital neuralgia. Vågå study of headache epidemiology. Cephalalgia. 2005;25:296–304.
6. Sjaastad O, Stolt-Nielsen A, Pareja JA, Fredriksen TA, Vincent M. Supraorbital neuralgia. On the clinical manifestations and a possible therapeutic approach. Headache. 1999;39:204–12.

Supratrochlear Nerve Block

Siddharth Chavali and Girija Prasad Rath

> **Key Points**
> - Both supraorbital and supratrochlear neuralgia may have similar presenting features
> - It is difficult to diagnose supratrochlear neuralgia in isolation
> - It is usually caused by compression along its course, possibly due to frowning or forced eye closure

Introduction

There has always been confusion regarding whether the symptoms of supraorbital neuralgia are caused by compressive lesions of the supraorbital nerve in isolation, or due to compression of the supraorbital and supratrochlear nerves in combination. Although these two nerves share the sensory innervation of the forehead, the supraorbital nerve is typically held accountable for neuralgic pain in this region. In a prospective study by Pareja and colleagues [1], pain was observed to be limited to the area supplied by the supratrochlear nerve. It offers insights on the best way to distinguish between supraorbital and supratrochlear neuralgia (Table 1).

S. Chavali · G. P. Rath (✉)
Department of Neuroanaesthesiology and Critical Care Neurosciences Centre,
All India Institute of Medical Sciences, New Delhi, India

G. P. Rath (ed.), *Handbook of Trigeminal Neuralgia*,
https://doi.org/10.1007/978-981-13-2333-1_11

Table 1 Difference between supraorbital and supratrochlear neuralgia

Supraorbital neuralgia	Supratrochlear neuralgia
Supraorbital nerve involved with or without involvement of supratrochlear nerve	Only supratrochlear nerve involved
Pain referred to whole forehead	Pain over medial forehead, extending to inner canthus of eye
Pain upon palpation of supraorbital notch	Pain upon palpation of medial one-third of supraorbital margin

The characteristics of supratrochlear neuralgia are as below:

- The pain is continuous or intermittent type.
- It is normally felt in the distribution of supratrochlear nerve, i.e. skin of lower forehead close to midline, pain may also cover the eyebrow and supero-internal angle of the orbit.
- Tenderness is usually present which can be elicited on palpation, at the point of emergence of the supratrochlear nerve, in the medial one-third of the superior orbital margin.
- Diagnosis is confirmed by pain relief after blockade of supratrochlear nerve.

Anatomy

The ophthalmic nerve which is a branch of trigeminal nerve provides sensory innervation to the scalp, forehead, upper eyelid, conjunctiva, and cornea. It also provides partial innervation to the nose, nasal mucosa, and meninges. Frontal nerve is the largest branch of ophthalmic nerve which enters the orbit via superior orbital fissure; it forms the supraorbital and supratrochlear nerves. As compared to the supraorbital nerve, the supratrochlear nerve is smaller and exits the orbit more medially, above the superior oblique muscle. The supratrochlear nerve is primarily responsible for sensation over the lower forehead near the midline, the conjunctiva, and the upper eyelid.

Etiopathogenesis of Supratrochlear Neuralgia

Supratrochlear neuralgia may occur spontaneously (idiopathic) or as a consequence of cranial trauma leading to local nerve damage, surgery, inflammation, or following varicella infection. Some of the idiopathic cases may be explained by compression of the nerve by other structures along its course. In the forehead, the supratrochlear nerve courses close to the calvarial surface, under the corrugator and frontalis muscles [2], and branches off into several nerves that may be compressed due to intramuscular entrapment. This mechanism may account pain that is triggered by frowning and forced eye closure.

Indications

- Pain relief for trigeminal neuralgia in ophthalmic division, usually in conjunction with supraorbital nerve blockade.
- Pain due to acute herpes zoster in ophthalmic division.
- Pain due to isolated supratrochlear neuralgia

Contraindications

- Uncooperative patient
- Any allergy or sensitivity to anesthetic agent
- Evidence of infection at the injection site
- Distortion of normal anatomical landmarks

Techniques

Landmark Guided (Classical Approach)

The supratrochlear nerve exits the orbit 1cm medial to the supraorbital nerve above the pulley of superior oblique muscle. Some authors suggest the nerve exiting via a supratrochlear foramen, although there is significant variability in the anatomy. As the supratrochlear foramen is difficult to be identified, the supraorbital foramen is used as a landmark which can be palpated along the supraorbital ridge.

- A 25-gauge intradermal needle may be used for the nerve block; it is introduced perpendicular to the skin 1cm medial to the supraorbital notch, between the notch and the bridge of the nose.
- Local anaesthetic (LA) solution (2–3 mL) can be injected in a fanlike distribution, after test aspiration.
- In case of paraesthesia, the needle should be withdrawn 1–2 mm before the LA is injected, in order to avoid intraneural injection.
- Some authors recommend placement of a roll of gauze under the orbital rim immediately after injection of LA. It prevents swelling of upper eyelid due to spread of LA through the loose alveolar tissue of the eyelid.

Ultrasound Guided

- The patient is asked to be seated for this block.
- The supraorbital notch on the affected side may be identified by palpation. The skin over the notch is prepared with antiseptic solution.

- A high frequency linear ultrasound transducer is placed in the longitudinal or transverse oblique position over the junction of supraorbital ridge and the bridge of nose.
- The supraorbital foramen can be identified as an interruption in the continuity of the hyper-echoic supraorbital ridge. The supratrochlear foramen may be identified in the same manner as for the supraorbital notch.
- A 25-gauge needle is advanced using an out-of-plane approach under continuous ultrasound guidance until the needle tip lies close to the supratrochlear foramen.

Drugs

- Commonly used LAs are lidocaine 1% or bupivacaine 0.25–0.5%.
- Lidocaine has a faster onset of action (3–5 min) and a duration of approximately 30–60 min.
- Bupivacaine has a slower onset of action (5 min) and a duration of approximately 4–5 h.
- Addition of sodium bicarbonate to the LA solution may reduce pain during injection of the drug and hasten onset of action.
- Addition of epinephrine (1:200,000) may increase the duration of the block
- Injection of a depot steroid may provide a longer duration of analgesia for neuropathic conditions.

Complications and Management

- The total dose of LA should be carefully titrated. Increased vascularity of the tissue in this area increases the risk of hematoma or ecchymosis formation.
- Infection may spread along the superior ophthalmic vein to the cavernous sinus with intracranial extension.
- Due to the presence of loose areolar tissue, pressure should be applied just below the infiltration site, to prevent swelling of eyelid.

Clinical Pearl

Infratrochlear neuralgia may present with paroxysmal or continuous pain in one of the three areas innervated by the infratrochlear nerve such as internal angle of the orbit and the medial upper eyelid, upper bridge of the nose, and/or the lacrimal caruncle [3, 4]. Pain is usually presented in association with tenderness on palpation of the infratrochlear nerve, above the internal canthus. The neuralgic pain gets relieved with anesthetic blockade of the infratrochlear nerve.

References

1. Pareja JA, López-Ruiz P, Mayo D, Villar-Quiles R-N, Cárcamo A, Gutiérrez-Viedma Á, Lastarria CP, Romeral M, Yangüela J, Cuadrado ML. Supratrochlear neuralgia: a prospective case series of 15 patients. Headache. 2017;57:1433–42.
2. Andersen NB, Bovim G, Sjaastad O. The frontotemporal peripheral nerves. Topographic variations of the supraorbital, supratrochlear and auriculotemporal nerves and their possible clinical significance. Surg Radiol Anat SRA. 2001;23:97–104.
3. Pareja JA, Casanova I, Arbex A, Cuadrado ML. Infratrochlear neuralgia. Cephalalgia Int J Headache. 2015;35:1202–7.
4. Villar-Quiles RN, García-Moreno H, Mayo D, Gutiérrez-Viedma Á, Ramos MI, Casas-Limón J, Cuadrado ML. Infratrochlear neuralgia: a prospective series of seven patients treated with infratrochlear nerve blocks. Cephalalgia. 2018;38:585–91.

Infraorbital Nerve Block

Siddharth Chavali and Girija Prasad Rath

Key Points

- Pain related to infraorbital neuralgia may be triggered by laughing or smiling due to compression on the infraorbital nerve
- It is difficult to diagnose infraorbital neuralgia which may be confused with maxillary sinusitis
- If nerve block is unsuccessful a field block with local anesthetic agent may be attempted

Introduction

The infraorbital nerve is the terminal branch of the maxillary nerve. It may become entrapped at any point along the length of its course, usually as it exits the skull via the infraorbital foramen causing shock-like unilateral pain its distribution known as ***infraorbital neuralgia***. The classical findings of infraorbital neuralgia include (1) Pain over upper cheek radiating to upper teeth, nose and upper eyelid usually described as sharp, tingling or electric-like; (2) Tenderness to pressure over infraorbital foramen with possible radiation of pain along the nerve distribution on the affected side; and (3) Symptoms may be exacerbated by smiling, laughing or excessive tension on the zygomatic muscles, possibly due to further compression of the infraorbital nerve.

S. Chavali · G. P. Rath (✉)
Department of Neuroanaesthesiology and Critical Care Neurosciences Centre,
All India Institute of Medical Sciences, New Delhi, India

G. P. Rath (ed.), *Handbook of Trigeminal Neuralgia*,
https://doi.org/10.1007/978-981-13-2333-1_12

Etiopathogenesis of Infraorbital Neuralgia

Infraorbital neuralgia is caused by entrapment of the infraorbital nerve, usually secondary to orbital fracture, trauma to the zygoma or teeth, complications after maxillary sinus surgery (Schluder's syndrome), infection or inflammation from maxillary sinusitis [1, 2]. It may be confused with maxillary sinusitis, periodontal disease or viral infections [3]. Diagnosis of infraorbital neuralgia is based on presenting symptoms and physical examination.

Anatomy

The maxillary nerve is the branch of the trigeminal ganglia that innervates the upper cheek. It exits the skull via the foramen rotundum, and continues along the sphenopalatine fossa where it enters the orbit via the inferior orbital fissure, and traverses the floor of the orbit within the infraorbital groove. It then exits the orbit via the infraorbital foramen, where it forms the infraorbital nerve. The infraorbital nerve is further divided into four branches such as inferior palpebral, internal nasal, external nasal, and superior labial branches which provides sensory innervation to the lower eyelid, lateral nares, upper lip, upper teeth, and gingiva. The infraorbital artery usually lies in close proximity to the nerve bundle. The infraorbital foramen is the usual site of nerve entrapment, followed by the maxillary sinus and zygoma (post-traumatic). Because the infraorbital artery has been found to be within the nerve bundle in 3/4th of previous cadaveric studies, any manoeuvre that increases arterial flow or pressure such as coughing, hypertension or head-down position may theoretically increase entrapment of the nerve within the foramen, causing exacerbation of pain symptoms.

Indications for Infraorbital Nerve Block

- Pain relief for trigeminal neuralgia in the maxillary distribution
- To provide postoperative analgesia in neonates and infants undergoing cleft lip repair
- Local anesthesia for surgeries of the lower eyelid/upper lip/endoscopic sinus surgery [4]

Contraindications

- Any allergy or sensitivity to anesthetic agent
- Evidence of infection at the injection site
- Distortion of normal anatomical landmarks
- Uncooperative patient

Techniques

Landmark Guided (Classical Approach)

For the classical landmark based technique, two approaches may be used, intraoral and extra-oral. A comparative study [5] suggested that there was no significant difference between the two approaches, even though the patients preferred the intraoral approach, subjectively. Regardless of the approach chosen, it is essential to ensure that the needle does not enter the infraorbital foramen; it reduces risk of injury to the globe. Palpation of the foramen throughout the procedure may help prevent inadvertent needle entry.

Intraoral Approach

- Topical anesthetic agents may be applied to the mucosa opposite the upper first premolar tooth.
- The patient is asked to look straight, and the mid-pupillary line should be imagined running down toward the inferior border of the infraorbital ridge.
- A finger should be kept in place over the inferior border of the infraorbital ridge throughout the procedure.
- The cheek should be retracted, and the needle should be introduced into the mucosa opposite the upper first premolar [6] approximately 5 mm from the buccal surface to a depth of about 15–20 mm, until it is palpated near the foramen.
- If the needle is extended too far superiorly/posteriorly, the orbit may be breached.
- After confirming negative aspiration for blood, 2–3 mL of local anesthetic solution may be injected.

Extraoral Approach (Fig. 1)

- The previously used landmarks may be used to identify the infraorbital foramen.
- A 25–27 G needle is advanced perpendicular to the skin with a cephalic and medial direction towards the foramen, piercing the skin, subcutaneous tissue and the quadratus labii superioris muscle, till bony resistance is encountered.
- A lateral to medial approach may reduce risk of penetration of the foramen due to the axis of the infraorbital foramen.
- Aspirate carefully, to ensure the needle is not placed intravascularly. Both the facial artery and vein lie in close proximity to the needle in this position. Due to the close proximity of the facial artery, use of vasoconstrictors should be avoided in the extra-oral approach to the nerve.
- After confirming negative aspiration, 1–3 mL of local anesthetic solution may be deposited, and gentle pressure should be applied to prevent hematoma formation.

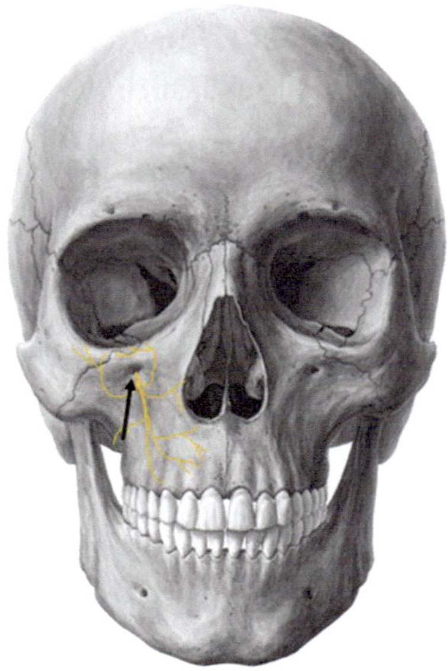

Fig. 1 Infraorbital nerve coming out of infraorbital foramen (site for the nerve block)

Ultrasound Guided (Fig. 2)

- The patient is asked to lie supine.
- The infraorbital foramen on the affected side may be identified by palpation. The skin over the notch should be prepared with antiseptic solution.
- A high frequency linear ultrasound transducer may be placed on the cheek just beside the nose, and slid cranially, to identify the dimple of infraorbital foramen, which will appear as a break in the continuity of the infraorbital ridge.
- Colour Doppler may be used to identify the exiting facial artery, accompanying the nerve.
- A 25-gauge needle is advanced using an out-of-plane approach under continuous ultrasound guidance until the needle tip lies close to the nerve. Spread of the anesthetic agent around the nerve may be visualized.

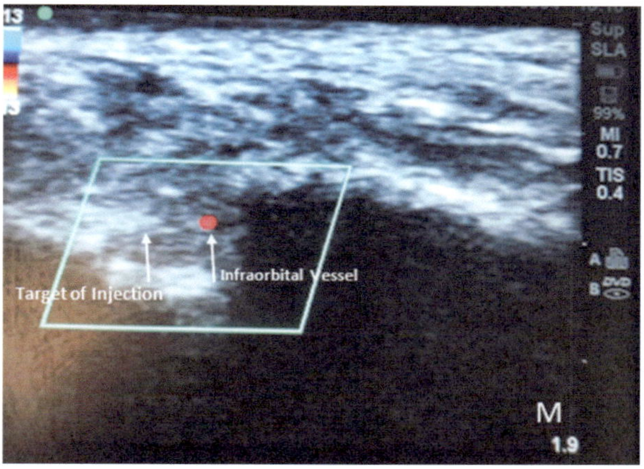

Fig. 2 Ultrasound guided infraorbital nerve block

Drugs

An infraorbital nerve block requires 1–3 mL of anesthetic agent.

- Lidocaine is the most commonly used agent. The onset of action is approximately 4–6 min, and the duration of effect is approximately 75 min.
- Bupivacaine is another frequently used anaesthetic agent. The onset of action of bupivacaine is slower, and the duration of anesthesia is about 4–8 times longer than that of lidocaine.
- The dose of anesthetic used in typical volumes for this procedure is not toxic.

Radiofrequency Treatment for Infra-Orbital Nerve

- Radiofrequency lesioning of the infraorbital nerve may also be considered in cases of refractory neuralgia, as it has proven effective in cases of idiopathic trigeminal neuralgia as well as herpes zoster of the trigeminal nerve.
- Heat radiofrequency lesioning could be a rational choice in the treatment of trigeminal neuralgia in elderly patients [7], but is usually accompanied by hypoesthesia or topoanesthesia.
- Pulsed radiofrequency lesioning has become more popular recently. Due to the interrupted nature of the pulsed output, sufficient time is allowed for the generated heat to dissipate, making this a non-neurodestructive technique.
- There are no reported cases of sensorimotor dysfunction related to pulsed radiofrequency therapy.
- There is a risk of skin ulceration during this procedure if the needle is positioned superficially. This can be avoided by inserting the electrode of the needle into the infraorbital canal. The probe tip temperature should be monitored throughout, to ensure that accidental penetration into the maxillary sinus has not occurred.

Complications and Management

- Small hematoma in the cheek which may disappear by a week
- Persistent paraesthesia of the upper lip. Hypoesthesia to touch and pain in the infraorbital region
- Hyperpathia, dysaesthesia, or double vision
- Intravascular injection into the facial artery/vein.
- Generalized seizures may occur with injection of even small intra-arterial volumes of local anesthetic, as arterial blood flow continues directly into the brain.
- Facial artery vasospasm
- Penetration of the infraorbital foramen may result in nerve damage by compression in the narrow space of the infraorbital canal
- Needle penetration of the orbital floor and damage to the globe.

Pearls

If the nerve block is unsuccessful, or if the location of the infraorbital notch is unclear, a field block may be attempted. Inject 5 mL of local anesthetic solution into the upper buccal margin in a fan-like distribution. Although this technique is not very accurate, it often achieves the same anesthetic effect.

References

1. Nam Y, Bahk S, Eo S. Anatomical study of the infraorbital nerve and surrounding structures for the surgery of orbital floor fractures. J Craniofac Surg. 2017;28:1099–104.
2. Hu KS, Kwak HH, Song WC, Kang HJ, Kim HC, Fontaine C, Kim HJ. Branching patterns of the infraorbital nerve and topography within the infraorbital space. J Craniofac Surg. 2006;17:1111–5.
3. Whittet HB. Infraorbital nerve dehiscence: the anatomic cause of maxillary sinus 'vacuum headache. Otolaryngol Head Neck Surg. 1992;107:21–8.
4. McAdam D, Muro K, Suresh S. The use of infraorbital nerve block for postoperative pain control after transsphenoidal hypophysectomy. Reg Anesth Pain Med. 2005;30:572–3.
5. Lynch MT, Syverud SA, Schwab RA, Jenkins JM, Edlich R. Comparison of intraoral and percutaneous approaches for infraorbital nerve block. Acad Emerg Med. 1994;1:514–9.
6. Jonnavithula N, Durga P, Kulkarni DK, Ramachandran G. Bilateral intra-oral, infra-orbital nerve block for postoperative analgesia following cleft lip repair in paediatric patients: comparison of bupivacaine vs bupivacaine-pethidine combination. Anaesthesia. 2007;62:581–5.
7. Rahman M, Richter EO, Osawa S, Rhoton AL. Anatomic study of the infraorbital foramen for radiofrequency neurotomy of the infraorbital nerve. Neurosurgery. 2009;64:423–8.

Auriculotemporal and Zygomaticotemporal Nerve Block

Siddharth Chavali and Girija Prasad Rath

Key Points

- Most common variant of trigeminal neuralgia (TGN) present with pain in the temple region
- There are two distinct presentations such as Auriculo-temporal neuralgia and Zygomatico-temporal syndrome
- Zygomatico-temporal neuralgia may mimic the features of Auriculo-temporal neuralgia

Introduction

Entrapment of the auriculotemporal nerve (ATN) could possibly be the most frequent of all the trigeminal headaches. Classically, the patient presents with complaints of headache in the area of temple. There are two main presentations when the ATN is involved: auriculotemporal neuralgia and auriculotemporal syndrome.

The **auriculotemporal neuralgia** usually presents with:

- Attacks of paroxysmal pain in preauricular/temple/retro-orbital regions, usually presenting at dawn [1]. The early morning headache seems to be associated with bruxism/jaw clenching during sleep.
- The patient may complain of auricular headache which may radiate to the temple.

S. Chavali · G. P. Rath (✉)
Department of Neuroanaesthesiology and Critical Care Neurosciences Centre, All India Institute of Medical Sciences, New Delhi, India

G. P. Rath (ed.), *Handbook of Trigeminal Neuralgia*,
https://doi.org/10.1007/978-981-13-2333-1_13

- Unilateral or bilateral headache may be associated with ear/parotid/jaw pain or numbness [2].
- The headache is throbbing type due to the close proximity of ATN to the temporal artery.
- Pain may be increased by talking/chewing/menses/palpation over the preauricular area, and it is a disorder which mainly affects middle-aged females [3].

The **auriculotemporal syndrome**, also called the **Frey syndrome** [4] is a complex of symptoms that includes flushing and unilateral hyperhidrosis over the ear and cheek. It occurs while eating or drinking anything that may stimulate saliva secretion from the parotid gland. These symptoms normally occur following parotid surgery or trauma to the gland [5] and there may be a concomitant trigeminal neuralgia (TGN). A possible mechanism could be improper regeneration of autonomic innervation of the parotid gland.

Anatomy

The mandibular division of the trigeminal nerve (V3) gives off three branches near the lateral pterygoid muscle: the auriculotemporal nerve (ATN), the inferior alveolar nerve and the lingual nerve. The ATN has a tortuous course, putting it at an increased risk of entrapment along its course. It is made up of two roots, which course around the middle meningeal artery, and then fuse to form a short trunk. The ATN runs to the medial side of the mandibular neck, then turns superiorly together with the superficial temporal artery, between the pinna and the mandibular condyle, under the parotid gland. After it exits the parotid gland, it arches over the zygomatic arch, and travels in front of the temporomandibular joint, till it pierces the temporalis muscle. It divides into five smaller branches: nerve to external auditory meatus, parotid branch nerve, anterior auricular nerve, auricular branch nerves, superficial temporal nerve which innervate the temporal region, temporomandibular joint, and the ear.

Etiopathogenesis of Auiculotemporal Neuralgia

Entrapment of the ATN may be due to spasm of the lateral pterygoid muscle or due to compression along its course between the medial and lateral pterygoid muscles; it causes facial numbness, mandibular pain or headaches [6]. It may also be trapped between the TMJ and muscles of mastication [7], or by the superficial temporal artery itself, possibly caused by intertwining of the nerve and artery.

Indications

- Pain relief for TGN in auriculotemporal distribution
- Pain relief for facial pain caused by TMJ anomalies

- Anesthesia for the external ear
- Pain relief for acute herpes zoster involving the external ear

Contraindications

- Any allergy or sensitivity to anesthetic agent
- Evidence of infection at the injection site
- Distortion of normal anatomical landmarks
- Uncooperative patient

Techniques of Auriculotemporal Nerve Block

Landmark Guided (Classical Approach)

- The patient lies supine with the head turned to opposite side from the side of block
- The temporal artery may be identified just above the origin of the zygoma
- A 25 G needle is inserted perpendicular to the skin just behind the superficial temporal artery until bony resistance is encountered
- Paraesthesia may be elicited, and after aspiration, 3 mL of anesthetic agent may be injected
- The needle may be then directed cephalad, and a further 2 mL of anesthetic is injected

Ultrasound Guided

- A high frequency linear probe may be placed transversely over the TMJ, and the superficial temporal artery is identified using colour Doppler
- The nerve looks like a small hyperlucent bundle adjacent to the artery
- The probe is then rotated to obtain a long-axis view tracking the nerve cephalad
- A 25 G needle is introduced using an out-of-plane approach to deliver the anesthetic solution

Zygomaticotemporal Neuralgia

The zygomaticotemporal nerve is a purely sensory branch of the maxillary division. It originates in the pterygopalatine fossa, enters the orbit through the inferior orbital fissure, and divides into zygomaticotemporal and zygomaticofacial branches. Then it passes along the inferolateral angle of the orbit, and enters into the temporal fossa through a bony canal in the zygomatic bone. This branch then ascends between the bone and the temporalis muscle. It pierces the deep temporal fascia approximately

2 cm above the zygomatic arch to innervate a small triangular area of skin in the temporal area.

The common site of entrapment along its course is when it crosses the zygomatic arch. The coronoid process usually moves cephalad in edentulous patients; it catches the nerve in the arch. The pain mimics the pattern of either observed in the ATN or maxillary nerve. The headache may become worse in the early morning after the dentures are removed the night before.

Technique of Zygomaticotemporal Nerve Block

- The patient is asked to lie supine, with the head turned away from affected side.
- The lateral orbital rim may be palpated at the level of the frontozygomatic suture.
- The index finger of the physician should be placed in the depression of the posterolateral aspect of the lateral orbital rim, inferior to the suture.
- The needle may be inserted just behind the palpating finger, and then 'walked down' the lateral orbital margin to the level of the lateral canthus.
- After confirming negative aspiration, 1–2 mL of anesthetic agent may be injected.

Drugs

- Commonly used local anesthetic agents are lidocaine 1% or bupivacaine 0.25–0.5%
- Alcohol, phenol or botulinum toxin have been used for the treatment of neuropathic pain, however, these agents are being used less frequently
- Injection of a depot steroid may provide a longer duration of analgesia for neuropathic conditions

Complications

- Hematoma due to close proximity of the superficial temporal artery
- Vascular injection of anesthetic agent
- Temporary facial nerve palsy may occur when the drug is injected at the level of the tragus, as the facial nerve courses along this point

Clinical Pearl

To avoid accidental facial nerve injury, an alternate approach may be considered during ATN block [8]. It utilizes a small volume of local anesthetic agent, and involves blockade of the nerve 1 cm above the tragus which is even further away from the route of facial nerve.

References

1. Murayama RA, Stuginski-Barbosa J, Moraes NP, Speciali JG. Toothache referred from auriculotemporal neuralgia: case report. Int Endod J. 2009;42:845–51.
2. Speciali JG, Gonçalves DAG. Auriculotemporal neuralgia. Curr Pain Headache Rep. 2005;9:277–80.
3. Trescot A. Headache: is it a migraine? Think again. Technol Reg Anesth Pain. 2005;9:68–72.
4. Motz KM, Kim YJ. Auriculotemporal syndrome (Frey syndrome). Otolaryngol Clin N Am. 2016;49:501–9.
5. Kamath RAD, Bharani S, Prabhakar S. Frey's syndrome consequent to an unusual pattern of temporomandibular joint dislocation: case report with review of its incidence and etiology. Craniomaxillofac Trauma Reconstr. 2013;6:1–8.
6. Komarnitki I, Andrzejczak-Sobocińska A, Tomczyk J, Deszczyńska K, Ciszek B. Clinical anatomy of the auriculotemporal nerve in the area of the infratemporal fossa. Folia Morphol (Warsz). 2012;71:187–93.
7. Schmidt BL, Pogrel MA, Necoechea M, Kearns G. The distribution of the auriculotemporal nerve around the temporomandibular joint. Oral Surg Oral Med Oral Pathol Oral Radiol Endod. 1998;86:165–8.
8. Bebawy JF, Bilotta F, Koht A. A modified technique for auriculotemporal nerve blockade when performing selective scalp nerve block for craniotomy. J Neurosurg Anesthesiol. 2014;26:271–2.

Mandibular Nerve Block for Trigeminal Neuralgia

Shiv Pratap Rana

Key Points

- Mandibular neuralgia is characterized by sharp shooting electric-shock like lower jaw pain triggered by chewing speaking and opening mouth
- Mandibular nerve block is used for the management of neuralgic pain in the distribution of the nerve in patients' refractory to medications
- The block may be performed on an outpatient setting; however, it is not free from complications

Introduction

Mandibular (V3) neuralgia is one of the most common causes of facial pain and it occurs in the distribution of the mandibular nerve which is the largest division of trigeminal nerve. Compression by a vascular loop around the mandibular portion of fifth nerve leading to paroxysmal painful attack in the face. The symptoms include unilateral, short-lived, severe, sharp, shooting, electric-shock like pains around the lower jaw. This pain may be triggered by innocuous stimuli such as eating, washing, shaving, and draughts of warm or cold air. Secondary causes may include cerebellopontine angle tumors and multiple sclerosis. Recently, it has been suggested that in some cases of temporomandibular joint syndrome, persistent idiopathic facial pain and myofascial pain syndrome may occur due to entrapment of the mandibular nerve.

S. P. Rana (✉)
Department of Anaesthesiology, Critical Care, and Pain Medicine, All India Institute of Medical Sciences (AIIMS), Bhopal, India

G. P. Rath (ed.), *Handbook of Trigeminal Neuralgia*,
https://doi.org/10.1007/978-981-13-2333-1_14

Anatomy

Mandibular branch of trigeminal nerve is a mixed nerve comprising of sensory and motor fibers. The nerve is formed by the large sensory branch arising from Gasserian ganglion, and a small motor branch arising from pons. The nerve then leaves the cranium through foramen ovale [1]. Mandibular nerve traverses anteriorly and inferiorly deep in to the infratemporal fossa just anterior to middle meningeal artery. Branches of mandibular nerve innervates cutaneous sensation to face, anterior two third of tongue, lower jaw, floor of mouth, lower lip, and motor fibers to the muscles of mastication [2, 3].

Indications

- Trigeminal neuralgia (TGN) involving lower jaw pain
- Acute intraoperative pain and trismus [2, 4]
- Surgical analgesia during carotid endarterectomy surgery [5, 6]
- Postoperative pain control after surgical reduction of a fractured mandible
- Chronic cancer pain involving lower jaw, floor of mouth and tongue.

Contraindication

- Acute inflammation at injection site
- Children and uncooperative patients
- Coagulopathy
- Known case of allergy to local anesthetics (LA)
- Distorted regional anatomy
- Fracture mandible

Drugs and Equipments

- Syringes: 3, 5, and 10 mL
- Needles: 26 G 1½ inch, 23 G 10 cm spinal needle
- Local anesthetics (LA): Lignocaine solution 2%
- Neurolytics: Absolute alcohol 100%, Phenol 6%, Dexamethasone
- Nerve stimulator, Radiofrequency (RF) generator, RF needle with 5 mm active tip

Techniques

Coronoid Approach

The patient is placed supine and routine monitors such as ECG, pulse oxymeter, and blood pressure are connected. The coronoid notch is localized by palpating the area below the zygoma by opening and closing the mouth. Lignocaine 1% is infiltrated to make skin wheal with a hypodermic needle. Through the coronoid (mandibular) notch, 23 G/10 cm spinal needle is advanced perpendicular to skin until it hit the lateral pterygoid plate. For precise localization of needle, C-arm image intensifier may be used; it helps confirming the needle position in antero-posterior and lateral views. Once bony structure is encountered, needle is withdrawn to 0.5–1 cm, and redirected posteriorly and inferiorly to about 1 cm further. The patient complaints of paraesthesia (Fig. 1); and there may be twitching of muscles of mastication when the nerve stimulator is used. LA solution 3–5 mL with or without steroids is injected for diagnostic block. For neurolytic blockade, 3–5 mL of 50–70% alcohol, or 6% phenol is injected [2, 3]. Continuous infusion of LA by catheter may be done in certain situations [7]. The procedure can be performed guided by ultrasonography, X-ray, or computed tomographic (CT) scan to avoid complications.

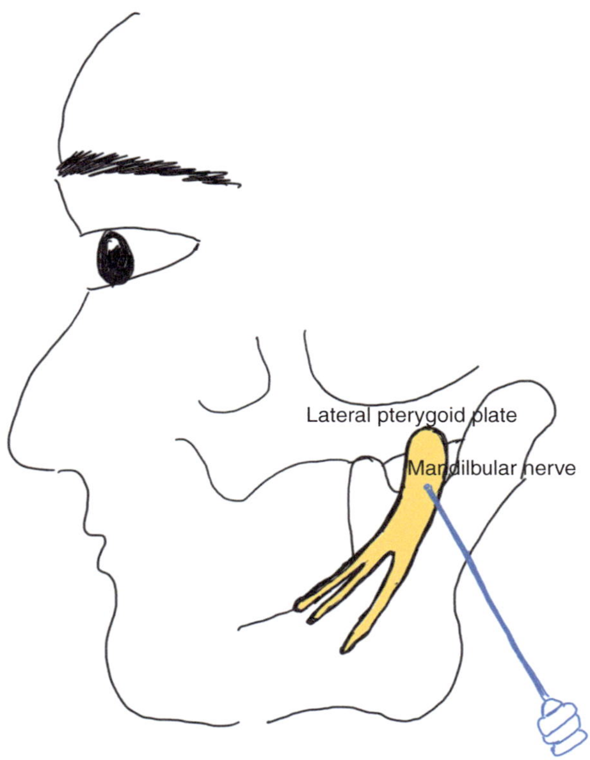

Fig. 1 Schematic diagram of Mandibular nerve block

Radiofrequency Ablation of Mandibular Nerve

Coronoid Approach

Pulsed radiofrequency (PRF) ablation of mandibular nerve can be done peripherally by coronoid approach. A RF needle of 10 cm length and 10 mm active tip is inserted similarly described above. After contacting lateral pterygoid plate with the RF needle, it is redirected posterior and inferiorly to get the muscle contraction of lower jaw. Sensory and motor stimulation are done at 50 and 2 Hz frequency to localise the nerve. If paraesthesia is obtained below 0.5 V stimulation, PRF ablation is done for 6 min duration at 42 °C [8].

Foramen Ovale Approach

Patient is positioned supine and all standard monitors connected. LA is infiltrated 2–3 cm lateral to angle of mouth. A RF needle of 10 cm length with 5 mm active tip is inserted under X-ray control in sub-mental view (Fig. 2) to the lateral portion of foramen ovale. Needle position is confirmed in lateral view to reach junction of petrous ridge and clivus. Sensory and motor stimulation are done at 50 and 2 Hz frequency to localize the nerve. If paraesthesia is obtained below 0.5 V stimulation, conventional (continuous) RF is done at 60–70 °C for 60–120 s [9].

Ultrasound-Guided Mandibular Nerve Block

Ultrasound has been used to block mandibular nerve for pain due to trismus [4]. The lateral pterygoid plate, the maxillary artery, and the pterygopalatine fossa can be seen by ultrasonography. Needle placement anterior to the lateral pterygoid plate,

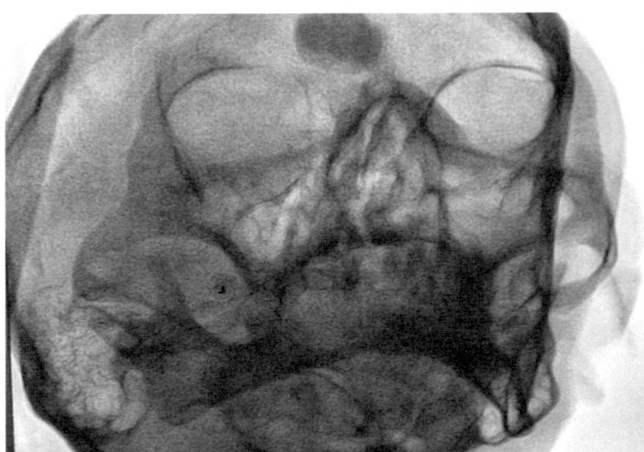

Fig. 2 Foramen ovale approach for mandibular nerve block

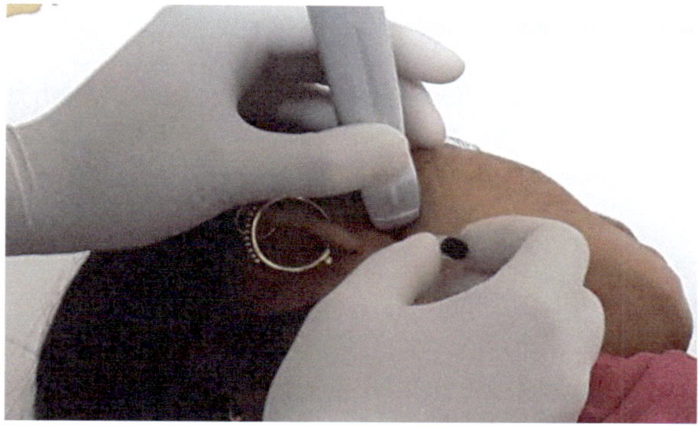

Fig. 3 Ultrasound guided mandibular nerve block

below the lateral pterygoid muscle, can be visualized in real-time ultrasonography and mandibular nerve is blocked (Fig. 3). This approach allows access to the pterygopalatine fossa and its contents [10].

CT-Guided Mandibular Nerve Block

Percutaneous technique of mandibular nerve block under CT-scan guidance is used for mandibular neuralgia or cancer pain. The foramen ovale is used as landmark on CT, and the mandibular nerve immediately caudal to the foramen ovale in the posterior margin of lateral pterygoid plate is the target site [11]. Rest of the technique is same as described above.

Complications [1, 12–14]

The following complications may occur following extra-oral mandibular nerve block. However, the procedure related complications may be avoided to a certain extent by using X-ray, ultrasound, CT scan or nerve stimulator.

- Local hematoma
- Masseter muscles weakness
- Needle track infection
- Inadvertent intravascular injection of LA and systemic toxicity thereof
- Increased pain after nerve block and dysesthesia
- Burning sensation, sensory loss, and numbness,
- Ataxia, vertigo, vasovagal syncope

Clinical Pearls

- It is important to insert the needle at least a depth of 5 cm to elicit paraesthesia for mandibular nerve. If no paraesthesia is reported, repositioning the needle is recommended.
- Aspiration of air during the block indicates needle entering the pharynx; it needs to be replaced and repositioned.

References

1. Warwick R, Williams PL, editors. Gray's anatomy British ed, vol. 35. Edinburgh: Churchill Livingstone; 1973.
2. Erdine S, Racz BG, Noe CE. Somatic blocks of the head and neck. In: Prithvi Raj P, et al., editors. Interventional pain management: image guided procedures. 2nd ed. Philadelphia, PA: Saunders Elsevier; 2008. p. 77–107.
3. Candido KD, Batra M. Nerve block of the head and neck. In: Benzon HT, Rathmell JP, Wu CL, Turk DC, Argoff CE, editors. Raj's Practical management of pain. 4th ed. Philadelphia, PA: Mosby Elsevier; 2008. p. 859–61.
4. Jain G, Yadav G, Singh AP, Singh Y, Singh DK. Efficacy of ultrasound-guided mandibular block in predicting safer anesthetic induction. Anesth Ess Res. 2016;10:184–8.
5. Bourke D, Thomas P. Mandibular nerve block in addition to cervical plexus block for carotid endarterectomy. Anesth Analg. 1998;87:1034–6.
6. Kavrut Ozturk N, Kavakli AS, Sagdic K, Inanoglu K, Umot Ayoglu R. A randomized controlled trial examining the effect of the addition of the mandibular block to cervical plexus block for carotid endarterectomy. J Cardiothorac Vasc Anesth. 2018;32:877–82.
7. Kohase H, Umino M, Shibaji T, Suzuki N. Application of a mandibular nerve block using an indwelling catheter for intractable cancer pain. Acta Anaesthesiol Scand. 2004;48:382–3.
8. Chua NHL, Halim W, Beems T, Vissers KC. Pulsed radiofrequency treatment for trigeminal neuralgia. Anesthesiol Pain Med. 2012;1:257–61.
9. Emril DR, Ho K-Y. Treatment of trigeminal neuralgia: role of radiofrequency ablation. J Pain Res. 2010;3:249–54.
10. Nader A, Bendok BR, Prine JJ, Kendall MC. Ultrasound-guided pulsed radiofrequency application via the pterygopalatine fossa: a practical approach to treat refractory trigeminal neuralgia. Pain Physician. 2015;18:E411–5.
11. Koizuka S, Saito S, Kubo K, Tomioka A, Takazawa T, Sakurazawa S, Goto F. Percutaneous radio-frequency mandibular nerve rhizotomy guided by CT fluoroscopy. AJNR Am J Neuroradiol. 2006;27:1647–8.
12. Sweet WH. Complications of treating trigeminal neuralgia: an analysis of the literature and response to questionnaire. In: Rovit RL, Murali R, Jannetta PJ, editors. Trigeminal neuralgia. Baltimore: Williams & Wilkins; 1990. p. 251–79.
13. Chaturvedi A, Dash HH. Prolonged vertigo and ataxia after mandibular nerve block for treatment of trigeminal neuralgia. J Anaesthesiol Clin Pharmacol. 2011;27:386–8.
14. Konishi R, Mitsuhata H, Akazawa S, Shimizu R. Temporary severe vertigo associated with mandibular nerve block with absolute alcohol for treatment of trigeminal neuralgia. Anesthesiology. 1997;87:699–700.

Maxillary Nerve Block for Trigeminal Neuralgia

Shiv Pratap Rana

Key Points

- Maxillary neuralgia is characterized by severe, sharp shooting upper jaw pain
- It is difficult to diagnose, and often mimics dental and facial pain
- Diagnostic, therapeutic, or neurolytic maxillary nerve blocks may be tried for management of the neuralgic pain

Introduction

Maxillary neuralgia is caused by the compression of second division of the trigeminal nerve arising from the ganglion either by a vascular loop or a tumor resulting in pain in upper jaw. Pain due to maxillary nerve compression is characterized by brief attacks of excruciating pain, usually described as being sharp shooting or electric in character, involving the distribution of maxillary nerve, namely the lower eyelid, cheeks, lateral nose, and upper lip. Painful attacks are triggered by jaw movement, smiling, chewing or speaking.

S. P. Rana (✉)
Department of Anaesthesiology, Critical Care, and Pain Medicine, All India Institute of Medical Sciences (AIIMS), Bhopal, India

G. P. Rath (ed.), *Handbook of Trigeminal Neuralgia*,
https://doi.org/10.1007/978-981-13-2333-1_15

Etiopathogenesis of Maxillary Neuralgia

Common causes of maxillary neuralgia are vascular loop around maxillary or trigeminal root entry zone (REZ), cerebellopontine angle tumor or idiopathic. Pain around the distribution of maxillary nerve is the clinical features of maxillary neuralgia. It may be confused with dental pain, maxillary sinusitis or sphenopalatine neuralgia.

Anatomy

Maxillary nerve is a pure sensory nerve, it exits the middle cranial fossa through the foramen rotundum and crosses the pterygopalatine fossa [2]. The different branches of second division supply sensation to upper jaw, dura, teeth, hard palate, soft palates, gums, and cheek (Fig. 1). The nerve finally emerges from the infraorbital foramen on the maxillary bone along with artery and vein. Any maneuver that stretches the mastication or pterygoid muscles causes painful attack in the area due to entrapment in the foramen or pressure over the nerve.

Indications

- Trigeminal neuralgia involving maxillary nerve
- Acute intraoperative pain during maxillofacial surgery
- Postoperative pain relief after maxillary surgery
- Cancer pain involving upper jaw

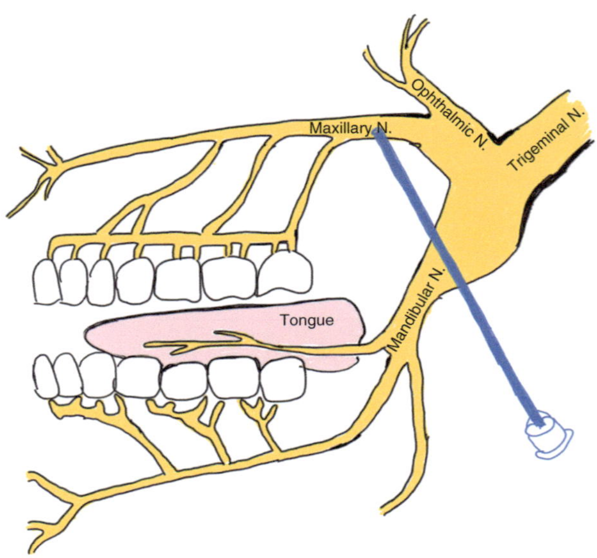

Fig. 1 Schematic diagram of maxillary nerve blockade

Contraindication

- Local infection at injection site
- Coagulopathy or patients on drugs which are known to alter hemostasis
- Patients with known allergy to local anesthetic agents
- Altered anatomy
- Refusal of patient

Drugs and Equipments

- Syringes: 3, 5, and 10 mL
- Needles: 26 G 1½, 23 G 10 cm spinal needle
- Local anesthetics: Lignocaine solution 2%
- Neurolytics: Absolute alcohol 100%, Phenol 6%, Dexamethasone
- Nerve stimulator

Techniques

There are mainly four approaches to block the second division i.e. maxillary nerve. Dentist prefer to do **intra-oral technique.** Rudolph Matas described an **Orbital approach** in which a needle is passed through the orbital cavity and it comes out of the infraorbital fissure [3]. An **anterolateral approach** was also used to block maxillary nerve with skin entry facing inferiorly to zygomatic arch and anterior to the coronoid process of the mandible [4]. **Lateral coronoid approach** first done by Levy and Baudoin in 1906 is more commonly done approach [5]. Currently, there are three techniques used to perform the maxillary nerve block: (a) High-tuberosity approach, (b) Greater palatine canal approach, and (c) Coronoid approach. The technique of extra-oral maxillary nerve block is described here.

Coronoid Approach

With patient in supine position, the coronoid notch is identified by asking the patient to open and close the mouth. A wheal is raised with 1% lignocaine local anesthetic (LA) solution. A needle is introduced at 2–2.5 cm anterior to external auditory meatus, and just below the zygomatic arch to skin to infiltrate with LA (Fig. 2). A 23 G spinal needle of 10 cm is advanced to hit the lateral pterygoid plate, and it would then be withdrawn 0.5–1 cm to position the needle anteriorly and superiorly at 45° towards root of nose (Fig. 1). Elicitation of paraesthesia is necessary to achieve a successful block. 3–5 mL of local anesthetic solution for diagnostic maxillary block, and 2–3 mL of 50–70% alcohol is used for neurolytic block. This technique can be done blindly (Fig. 2), X-ray guided (Fig. 3), CT-guided or nerve stimulator-guided approaches [6]. Pulsed radiofrequency (PRF) ablation of

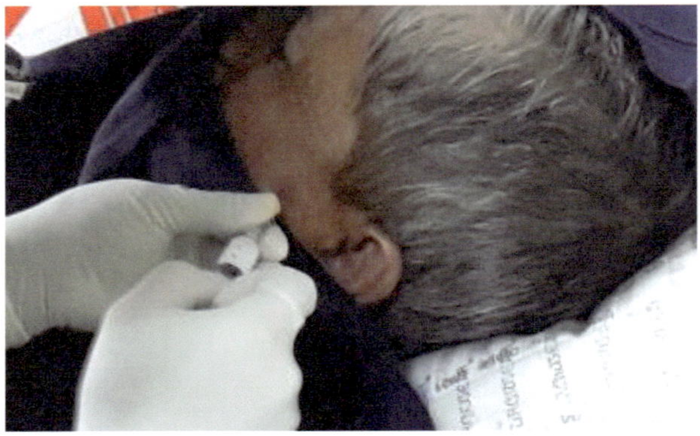

Fig. 2 Lateral coronoid approach for maxillary nerve block

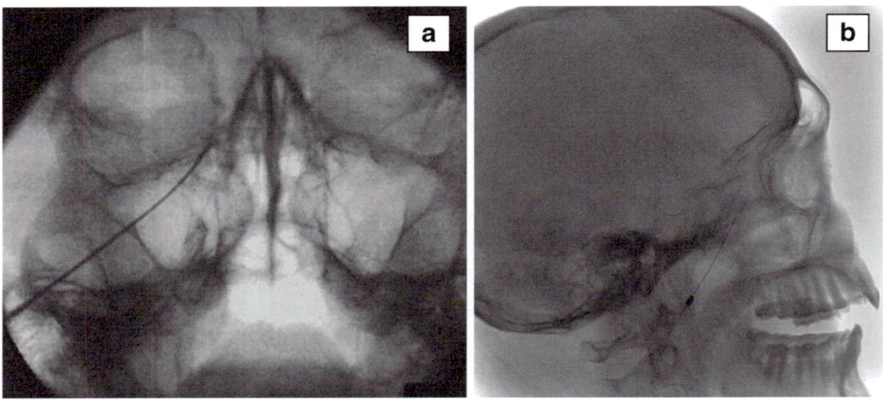

Fig. 3 X-ray guided maxillary nerve block; anteroposterior (**a**) and lateral (**b**) view shows needle in the pterygopalatine fossa (With permission, Serdar Erdine. Interventional Pain Management: Image guided procedures)

maxillary nerve can be done using 5 mm active tip, 10 cm long RF needle for 5–10 min after sensory (50 Hz, 0.2–0.5 V) and motor (2 Hz) stimulation [1]. The patient is closely observed in recovery area to observe pain in the orbit or other complications, if any.

Ultrasound Guided Maxillary Nerve Block

Ultrasound imaging is safe and simple non-invasive method to localise the maxillary nerve along the maxillary artery (Fig. 4). A 6–13 MHz frequency linear probe or hockey stick probe is used to block the maxillary nerve in the sphenopalatine fossa [7]. Local anaesthetic 4–5 mL combined with steroid is placed below the lateral pterygoid muscle; it results in immediate pain relief due to blockade of maxillary nerve (Fig. 5) [8]. Ultrasonography guided procedures help in the visualization

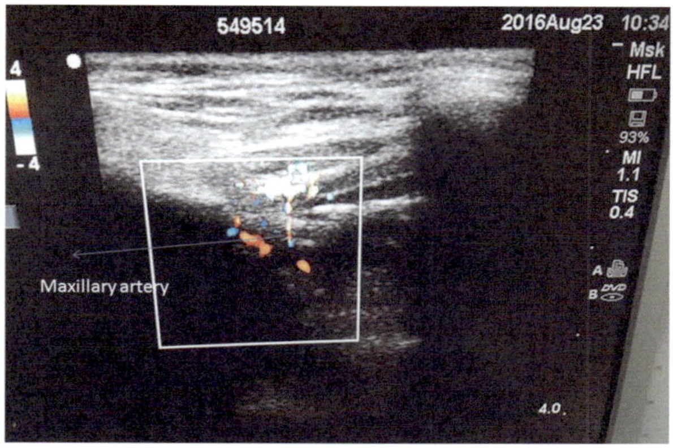

Fig. 4 Ultrasound guided for maxillary nerve block

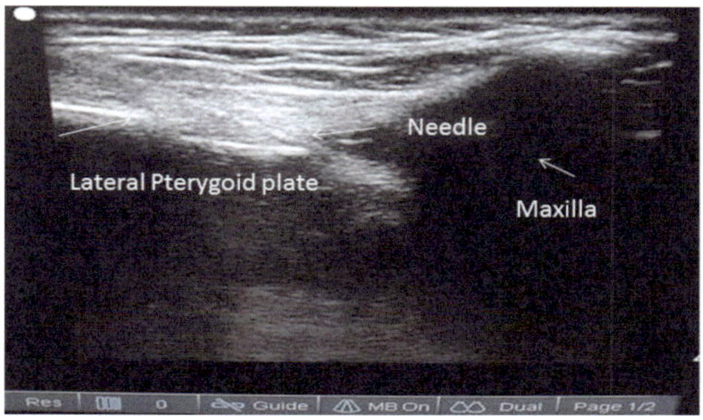

Fig. 5 Ultrasound image shows needle in the pterygopalatine fossa for maxillary nerve block

of vascular structures, such as maxillary artery, and hence, an accidental intravascular injection of the drug can be prevented. Radiation hazards are also avoided with using ultrasonography.

Complications [1, 9]

- Cheek swelling, orbital swelling, and local hematoma
- Parasthesia and numbness due to trauma to the maxillary nerve
- Inadvertent blockade of nerves near maxillary nerve
  - Sixth cranial nerve blockade causing diplopia
  - Transient blockade of facial nerve
  - Optic nerve blockade: Rare, may lead to temporary blindness
  - Retrobulbar nerve blockade
- Inadvertent IV injection of drugs and LA toxicity
- Infection in the needle track
- Allergic and vaso-vagal reactions

Clinical Pearls

- Vascular puncture and hematoma formation are common in maxillary nerve block which can be prevented with the use of ultrasonography.
- Aspiration of air during the block indicates needle entering the pharynx and the needle needs replaced and repositioned.

References

1. Erdine S, Racz BG, Noe CE. Somatic blocks of the head and neck. In: Prithvi Raj P, et al., editors. Interventional pain management: image guided procedures. 2nd ed. Philadelphia, PA: Saunders Elsevier; 2008. p. 77–107.
2. Warwick R, Williams PL, editors. Gray's Anatomy, British Ed. 35. Edinburgh: Churchill Livingstone; 1973.
3. Allen CW. Local and regional anesthesia. Philadelphia: WB Saunders; 1915.
4. Schlosser H. Erfahrungen in der Neuralgiebehandlung mit Alkoholeinspritzungen: Verhandl. D Cong Finnere Med. 1907;24:49.
5. Levy F, Baudoin A. Les injections profondes dans le traitment de la neuralgie. Presse Med. 1906;13:108.
6. Okuda Y, Okuda K, Shinohara M, Kitajima T. Use of computed tomography for maxillary nerve block in the treatment of trigeminal neuralgia. Reg Anesth Pain Med. 2000;25:417–9.
7. Tsui BC. Ultrasound imaging to localize foramina for superficial trigeminal nerve block. Can J Anaesth. 2009;56:704–6.
8. Nader A, Kendall MC, De Oliveria GS, Chen JQ, Vanderby B, Rosenow JM, Bendok BR. Ultrasound-guided trigeminal nerve block via the pterygopalatine fossa: an effective treatment for trigeminal neuralgia and atypical facial pain. Pain Physician. 2013;16:E537–45.
9. Sweet WH. Complications of treating trigeminal neuralgia: an analysis of the literature and response to questionnaire. In: Rovit RL, Murali R, Jannetta PJ, editors. Trigeminal neuralgia. Baltimore: Williams & Wilkins; 1990. p. 251–79.

Mental Nerve Block

Siddharth Chavali and Girija Prasad Rath

Key Points

- Mental nerve neuralgia is also known as Numb Chin Syndrome
- May be a sentinel feature of malignant carcinomas
- Direct injection into the mental foramen may cause compressive damage of mental nerve

Introduction

Mental nerve neuralgia is a painful disorder in the distribution of the mental nerve. The first description of mental nerve neuropathy was given by Charles Bell in 1830, who reported the phenomenon in a patient with advanced breast cancer due to a bony metastasis in her left mandible [1]. Mental nerve neuropathy, which has also been called **Numb Chin Syndrome** is a purely sensory neuropathy identified by paraesthesia or numbness in the lower lip and chin. The clinical presentations are paraesthesia (tingling/burning/pins and needles) localised to a discrete area of the lower maxillary/mandibular region of the face, patients experiences a numb/swollen lower lip, loss of sensitivity may lead to inadvertent biting, or injury to the lower lip, symptoms are predominantly unilateral; however bilateral symptoms may also be present [2].

S. Chavali · G. P. Rath (✉)
Department of Neuroanaesthesiology and Critical Care Neurosciences Centre, All India Institute of Medical Sciences, New Delhi, India

G. P. Rath (ed.), *Handbook of Trigeminal Neuralgia*,
https://doi.org/10.1007/978-981-13-2333-1_16

Etiopathogenesis of Mental Nerve Neuralgia

Etiology may be local or systemic, and the most common mechanisms of nerve injury are mechanical or chemical modalities. Mechanical injury may involve traction, compression or resection of the nerve, possibly due to trauma or surgery. Chemical damage to the mental nerve can occur either from local irrigation with neurotoxic chemicals during dental surgery, or due to immunological response of the body to infection [3]. Mental nerve neuropathy may also be a harbinger for metastatic carcinomas, and any patient presenting with such symptoms should undergo a comprehensive workup for any malignancies [4–6]. Metastatic lesions to the mandible causing compression of either the mental or inferior alveolar nerve are thought to be the reason for neuropathic symptoms.

Anatomy

Sensory innervation to the face is provided by the trigeminal nerve, which branches into the ophthalmic (V1), maxillary (V2) and mandibular (V3) nerves. The mandibular division of the trigeminal nerve (V3) gives rise to three branches at the level of the lateral pterygoid muscle: the auriculotemporal nerve, the inferior alveolar nerve (IAN) and the lingual nerve. The IAN descends in the pterygoid fascia between the medial pterygoid muscle and the mandibular ramus, running postero-laterally to the lingual nerve, before entering the mandibular foramen. The IAN then courses along the inferior surface of the mandible till the mental foramen. At the level of the mental foramen, which lies approximately at the second premolar tooth, the IAN divides into the mental nerve, which exits the mental foramen along with blood vessels, and the incisive nerve, which continues along the interior aspect of the mandible (Fig. 1).

The mental nerve then courses superficially, and divides into three sensory branches behind the depressor anguli oris muscle: one innervating the skin of the mental area, and the other two innervating the skin of the lower lip and the gingiva up to the second premolar. An accessory mental nerve and foramen have been recently identified as a cause of unanticipated mental nerve damage [7]. It has been suggested that any surgical procedures involving the anterior mandible should be preceded by a computed tomographic (CT) scan of the jaw. A difference in the size of the left and right mental foramina could indicate the presence of an accessory mental foramen.

Indications for Mental Nerve Block

- Pain relief for trigeminal neuralgia in mental nerve distribution.
- Anesthesia for dental procedures
- Anesthesia for lower lip/chin

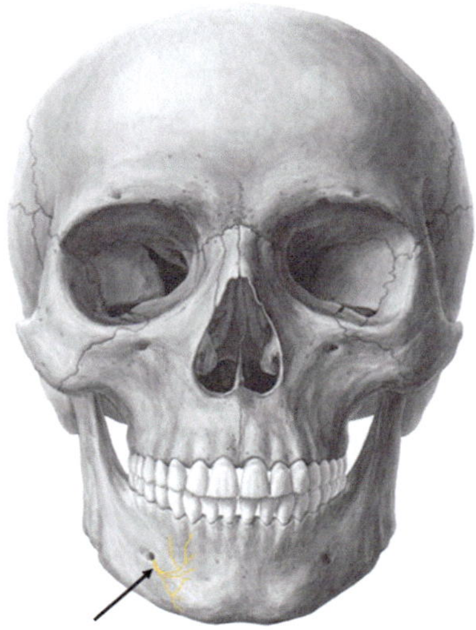

Fig. 1 Mental nerve coming out of mental foramen (site for the nerve block)

Contraindications

- Any allergy or sensitivity to anesthetic agent
- Evidence of infection at the injection site
- Distortion of normal anatomical landmarks
- Uncooperative patient

Techniques

Landmark Guided (Classical Approach)

Similar to infraorbital nerve blockade, both intraoral and extra-oral approaches to the blockade of the mental nerve have been described. For both blocks, the patient is asked to be seated or lie supine.

Extra-Oral Approach

- The mental foramen is located along the mid-pupillary line on the mental process of the mandible, in proximity to the inferior premolar tooth.
- A 25/27 G needle is inserted perpendicular the skin 1 cm lateral to the foramen palpated.
- The needle is directed in a lateral to medial direction to avoid penetration of the mental foramen.

- The needle should be withdrawn immediately if the patient reports paraesthesia, indicating accidental foraminal entry.
- After negative aspiration for blood, 1.5–3 mL of anesthetic solution may be injected slowly.

Ultrasound Guided Pulsed Radiofrequency

- Ultrasound imaging may be used to identify the mental foramen accurately, since it may be difficult to identify it through palpation alone.
- The mental foramen is localised by scanning transversely in a cephalad direction from the inferior border of the mandible using a 10–12 MHz linear transducer.
- The mandible appears as a hyperechoic linear structure, and the mental foramen is visualized as a hypoechoic cleft within this structure. The exiting vascular structures may be identified using Doppler (Fig. 2).
- The needle may be inserted using an in-plane approach, until it is seen entering the mental foramen.
- A pulsed radiofrequency current of 45 V lasting 2 min is then administered, with the maximum temperature not exceeding 42 °C

Intraoral Approach

- The mental foramen is identified using the landmarks described above.
- The lower lip is retracted, and topical anesthetic is applied to the inferior labial sulcus at the base of the first inferior premolar tooth.
- A finger should be kept just below the mental foramen throughout the procedure, to avoid accidental penetration of the mental foramen.
- A 25/27 G needle may be directly anteriorly and inferiorly toward the palpating finger to a depth of approximately 1 cm.
- After negative aspiration for blood, 1.5–3 mL of anesthetic solution may be injected.

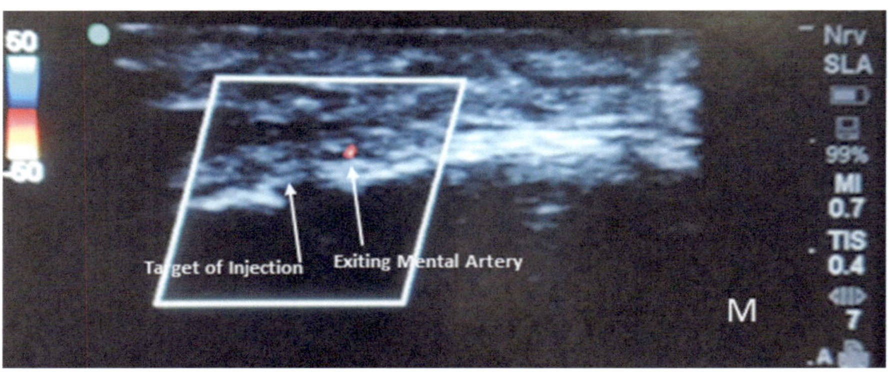

Fig. 2 Ultrasound guided mental nerve block

Slow injection of anesthetic agents has been reported to be more comfortable to patients, and the intraoral approach is subjectively better tolerated than the percutaneous approach.

Drugs

- Commonly used local anesthetic agents are lidocaine 1% or bupivacaine 0.25–0.5%.
- Alcohol, phenol or botulinum toxin have been used to treat neuropathic pain, however these agents are being used less frequently.
- Injection of a depot steroid may provide a longer duration of analgesia for neuropathic conditions.

Complications and Management

- Direct injection into the mental foramen may cause compressive damage to the mental nerve and lead to neurapraxia
- Vascular injection of anesthetic agent
- Hematoma
- Infection

Clinical Pearl

If the mental foramen is not directly palpable, the local anesthetic may be injected into the buccal mucosa between the two inferior premolar teeth to ensure a similar block.

References

1. Furukawa T. Charles Bell's description of numb chin syndrome. Neurology. 1988;38:331.
2. Laurencet FM, Anchisi S, Tullen E, Dietrich PY. Mental neuropathy: report of five cases and review of the literature. Crit Rev Oncol Hematol. 2000;34:71–9.
3. Di Lenarda R, Cadenaro M, Stacchi C. Paresthesia of the mental nerve induced by periapical infection: a case report. Oral Surg Oral Med Oral Pathol Oral Radiol Endod. 2000;90:746–9.
4. Requena A, Riera-Mestre A, Formiga F, Vidaller A, Pujol R. Metastatic prostate carcinoma presenting as numb chin syndrome in elderly people. J Am Geriatr Soc. 2008;56:581–2.
5. Sasaki M, Yamazaki H, Aoki T, Ota Y, Sekiya R, Kaneko A. Bilateral numb chin syndrome leading to a diagnosis of Burkitt's cell acute lymphocytic leukemia: a case report and literature review. Oral Surg Oral Med Oral Pathol Oral Radiol Endod. 2011;111:e11–6.
6. Zadik Y, Benoliel R, Fleissig Y, Casap N. Painful trigeminal neuropathy induced by oral bisphosphonate-related osteonecrosis of the jaw: a new etiology for the numb-chin syndrome. Quintessence Int Berl Ger. 2012;1985(43):97–104.
7. Gupta S, Soni JS. Study of anatomical variations and incidence of mental foramen and accessory mental foramen in dry human mandibles. Natl J Med Res. 2012;2:28–30.

Intra-Oral Nerve Blocks for Trigeminal Neuralgia

Rahul Yadav and Siddharth Chavali

Key Points

- Intraoral nerve blocks for management for trigeminal neuralgia (TGN) are associated with excellent short-term results
- Few of these nerve blocks are good alternatives to peripheral nerve blocks for TGN carried out with extra-oral approaches
- There is always a possibility of the patients undergoing multiple episodes of injection after intraoral block

Introduction

The management of drug-resistant trigeminal neuralgia (TGN) includes peripheral injections of different chemical agents into the affected nerve. Historically, chloroform was the first substance used for this purpose. Later on, substances like glycerol, phenol, boiling water, high concentrations of tetracaine [1], and streptomycin [2, 3] were also used. Alcohol injections [4] are preferred at the initial presentation of TGN or in elderly

R. Yadav (✉)
Oral and Maxillofacial Surgery, Centre for Dental Education and Research (CDER), All India Institute of Medical Sciences (AIIMS), New Delhi, India

S. Chavali
Department of Neuroanaesthesiology and Critical Care, All India Institute of Medical Sciences (AIIMS), New Delhi, India

G. P. Rath (ed.), *Handbook of Trigeminal Neuralgia*,
https://doi.org/10.1007/978-981-13-2333-1_17

Table 1 Intra-oral blocks involving mandibular and maxillary nerves

Blockade of mandibular nerve and branches	Blockade of maxillary nerve and branches
Mental nerve block Inferior alveolar nerve block Buccal nerve block Lingual nerve block Mandibular nerve block	Infraorbital or anterior superior alveolar nerve block Posterior superior alveolar nerve block Maxillary nerve block

patients with similar problem [5]. Patients with significant medical co-morbidities who are not fit to undergo invasive surgeries safely, may also benefit from alcohol injection [5]. Peripheral alcohol nerve block is associated with a variable duration of pain relief ranging from 6 to 16 months [6]. There are two distinct techniques described for peripheral nerve blocks for TGN: (a) extra-oral or percutaneous nerve blocks and (b) intraoral nerve block; this chapter will focus on intraoral nerve block techniques involving mandibular and maxillary nerves, and their branches (Table 1). The preferred local anesthetic (LA) agents include lignocaine (1–2%) and bupivacaine (0.5%) with or without adrenaline (1:2,00,000). Currently, the use of ropivacaine (0.5%) has also been increased as it has minimal cardiovascular risks with a prolonged duration of action.

Indications

- Diagnostic and therapeutic blocks for TGN with LAs
- Maxillary and mandibular trauma
- Dento-alveolar surgeries
- Post-extraction pain

Contraindications

- Hypersensitivity or allergy to LAs
- Bleeding disorders or coagulopathies
- Distorted anatomical landmarks for peripheral blocks
- Presence of cardiac diseases
- Uncooperative patients

Blockade of Mandibular Nerve and Branches

Mental Nerve Block

Area anesthetized: Ipsilateral lower lip, buccal tissue anterior to mental foramen, and skin of chin.

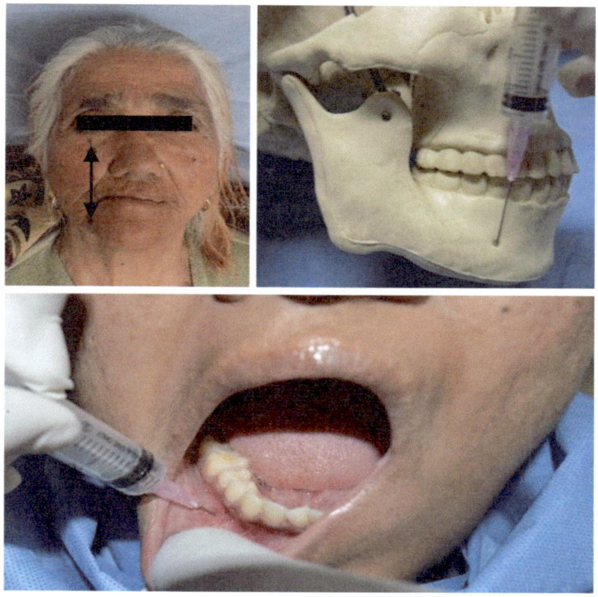

Fig. 1 (Clockwise): An imaginary line passing through the pupil, infra orbital foramen, corner of mouth and mental foramen; Identifying the mental foramen with needle which lies between the root apices of premolars and approximately twice the height of crown of premolar apically; Intra-oral mental nerve block

Technique

- The patient is asked to close mouth with relaxed lips and look forward.
- An imaginary line passing through supraorbital notch, pupil of eye, infraorbital notch, towards the inferior border of mandible should pass through mental foramen (Fig. 1).
- Index finger is placed in mandibular labial vestibule and the lip reflected laterally; needle is inserted in the midway between gingival crest and inferior border of mandible in line with the imaginary line passing between the bicuspids in antero-inferior direction to enter the foramen.
- LA 1 mL followed by 0.5 mL of absolute alcohol is injected.

Inferior Alveolar Nerve Block

Area anesthetized: Body of the mandible and mandibular teeth, mucous membrane, and structures anterior to the first mandibular molar.
Technique

- Patient is asked to open the mouth wide on sitting position, and the mucobuccal fold is palpated posteriorly over the external oblique ridge (Fig. 2).
- Thumb is moved over the anterior border of mandible to palpate the deepest portion on anterior border of ramus i.e., coronoid notch.

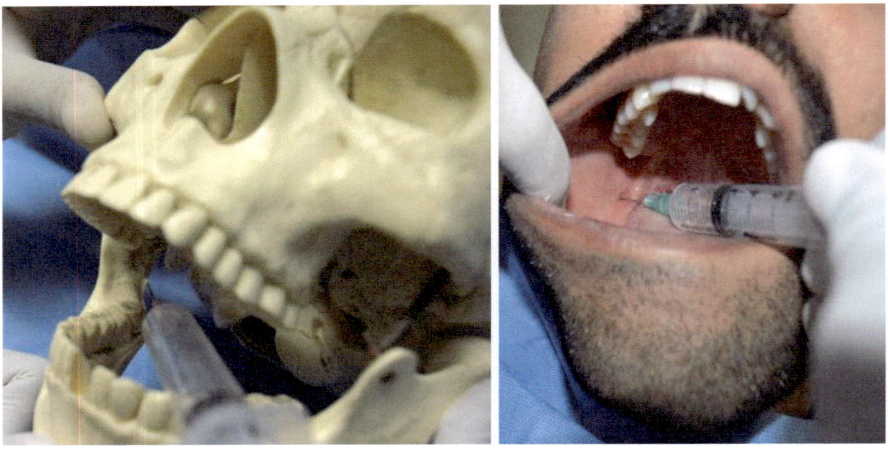

Fig. 2 (Clockwise): Inserting the needle in pterygomandibular space near the mandibular foramen, directing from the opposite side of premolars, Intra-oral inferior alveolar nerve block

- Thumb is then moved over the internal oblique ridge in line with the coronoid notch and simultaneously holding the posterior border of mandible extra-orally with the index finger of left hand, thus having an approximate idea of the width of the mandibular ramus, as the area of insertion of needle i.e. the mandibular foramen is approximately just in the middle of the total antero-posterior width of mandibular ramus.
- A 25 G needle is inserted from opposite side premolar region parallel to the mandibular occlusion plane keeping in mind the area of insertion; approximately 20–25 mm of the needle will be inserted in soft tissue.
- Care should be taken if bone is encountered prematurely, the direction of the syringe is to be changed in that condition, towards the mid-sagittal plane. Similarly, if no bony contact is made even after excessive insertion of needle, the direction of needle needs to be changed accordingly away from the sagittal plane i.e. towards the contralateral molar teeth. This is to counter the variations in mediolateral ramus flare in different individuals.
- After bone is contacted at an appropriate distance, 2 mL of LA is injected followed by injection of 0.8 mL of absolute alcohol for neurolysis.

Lingual Nerve Block

Areas anesthetized: Ipsilateral anterior two thirds of the tongue and floor of the oral cavity, mucosa and ipsilateral mucoperiosteum on lingual side of mandible.
Technique: Like inferior alveolar nerve block

Blockade of Maxillary Nerve and Branches

Anterior Superior Alveolar or Infra-Orbital Nerve Block

Area Anesthetized: Ipsilateral lower eyelid, lateral aspect of nose and upper lip
Technique

- Patient is asked to open the mouth and look forward.
- The muco-buccal fold is palpated just superior to first maxillary premolar with the help of thumb. Infra orbital foramen is palpated with the index finger which guides the needle accordingly (Fig. 3).
- An imaginary line connecting the supraorbital notch, pupil and corner of mouth passes through the infraorbital foramen.
- Using a 25 G needle, inject around 1 mL of LA followed by 0.5 mL of absolute alcohol after negative aspiration.

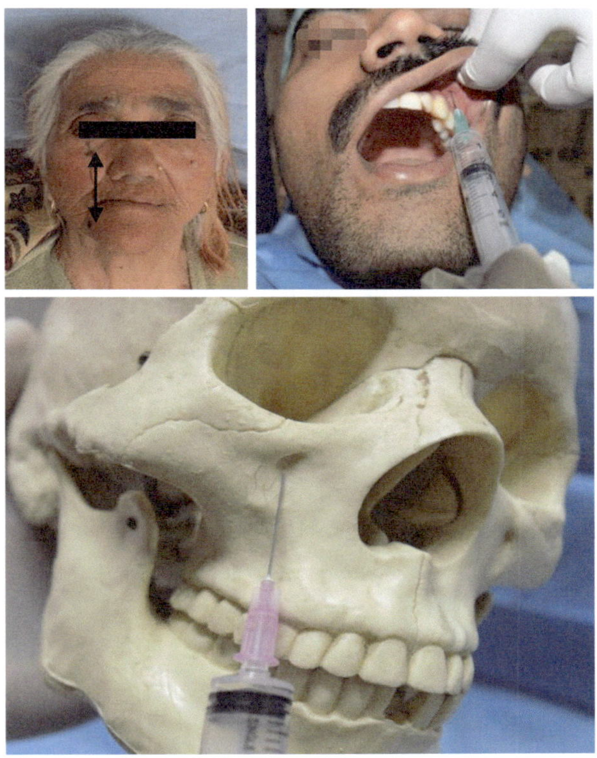

Fig. 3 (Counterclockwise): Locating the infra orbital foramen through the imaginary line; Inserting the needle in infraorbital foramen keeping the syringe in line and parallel to the first premolar and pupil of eye; Intra-oral infraorbital nerve block on left side

Posterior Superior Alveolar Nerve Block

Area Anesthetized: Maxillary molar region and overlying soft tissues
Technique

- The patient is asked to open mouth partially—the muco-buccal fold is palpated with the thumb of left hand and soft tissue is retracted laterally opposite the second maxillary molar, palpating the zygomatico-maxillary buttress region (Fig. 4)
- Needle is inserted at the muco-buccal fold opposite the maxillary second molar bisecting the tooth with direction of insertion being 45° to the maxillary occlusal plane going medially towards the midline and backwards.
- The needle is advanced slowly, and is withdrawn and retracted slightly, in case of resistance until the needle inserted approximately 20 mm.
- After negative aspiration 2 mL of LA injcted followed by injection of absolute alcohol 0.8 mL.
- Depth of needle insertion should be kept in mind; over insertion can lead to injury to pterygoid venous plexus or internal maxillary artery, leading to hematoma formation
- If hematoma occurs, apply pressure against the zygomatico-maxillary buttress and apply cold packs and start empirical antibiotics for 3–5 days.

Intra-Oral Maxillary Nerve Block

Area Anesthetized: Ipsilateral maxillary teeth, bone and soft tissue, some part of soft palate, lower eyelid, cheek, side of nose and upper lip

There are two techniques described for intra-oral maxillary blockade: **(a) High tuberosity technique and (b) Greater palatine canal approach**.

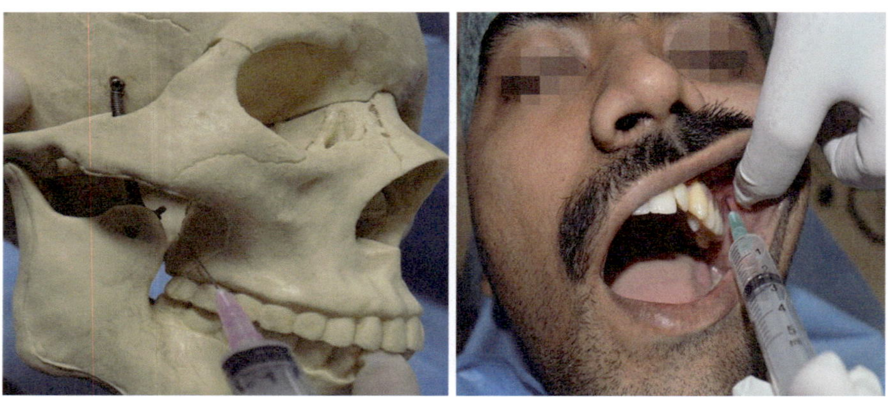

Fig. 4 Inserting the needle 45° to maxillary occlusal plane, bisecting the second molar and going medially towards the midline and backwards for posterior superior alveolar nerve block; Posterior superior alveolar nerve block on left side

Advantages: High success rate with minimum number of needle pricks for anesthesia on ipsilateral maxilla; less traumatic.

Disadvantages: As there are no bony landmarks available, technique is arbitrary and over insertion may occur. In greater palatine approach, there could be bony obstructions in canal in approximately 15 % of cases which makes it very difficult to negotiate. There is also a risk of hematoma with this block.

- High Tuberosity Technique
  - The area of interest is superior and medial to posterior superior alveolar nerve i.e. maxillary nerve as it passes through the pterygopalatine fossa. For this, a 25 G long needle of length approximately 32 mm is required.
  - Similar technique as utilized for posterior superior alveolar nerve block is followed.
  - Patient is asked to open mouth partially; the mucobuccal fold is palpated with the thumb of left hand and soft tissue is retracted laterally opposite the second maxillary molar, palpating the zygomatico-maxillary buttress region.
  - A 25 G needle of length 32 mm is inserted at the muco-buccal fold opposite the maxillary second molar bisecting the tooth with the direction of insertion 45° to the maxillary occlusal plane going medially towards the midline and backwards
  - If any resistance is felt during slow advancement of the needle it must be withdrawn slightly and adjusted to re-direct more backwards till the needle inserted 30 mm; at this length the needle approximates the maxillary nerve in pterygopalatine fossa.
  - After negative aspiration 2 mL of LA is injected, followed by injection of absolute alcohol 0.8 mL.
- Greater Palatine Canal Approach
  - A 25 gauge long (32 mm) needle is required.
  - Greater palatine foramen can be located by inserting the needle from opposite side, around 1 cm palatally to the crest of palatal gingiva between the second and third maxillary molars. A shallow depression can be palpated at this site and accordingly will guide the needle in greater palatine foramen (Fig. 5).
  - Needle should be inserted slowly; there can be bony interferences once a length of 30 mm is inserted, the needle tip would lie in the pterygopalatine fossa.
  - LA 2 mL is injected followed by 0.8 mL of absolute alcohol.

Complications After Intraoral Blocks

- **Trismus and swelling** are most common complication; easily managed with prophylactic antibiotics and anti-inflammatory medications
- **Necrosis of overlying mucosa and soft tissue**: Injection of recommended quantities of alcohol in vicinity of the foramen may prevent these rare complications. The management includes local debridement, maintenance of oral hygiene, and symptomatic treatment to relieve pain

- **Necrosis in fascial spaces of head and neck with superseded infection** may occur very rarely (Fig. 6). It may require aggressive treatment if patency of airway is threatened with tracheostomy along with therapeutic antibiotics.

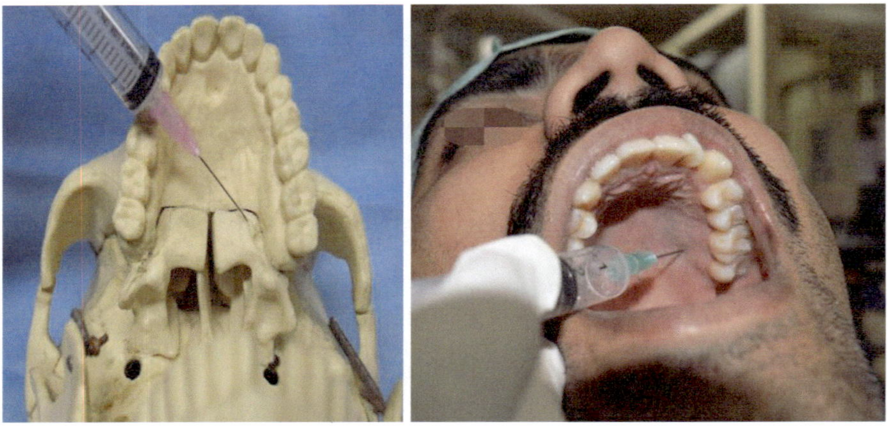

Fig. 5 Inserting the needle in greater palatine foramen approximately 1 cm from palatal gingival crest towards the midline, and between second and third maxillary molars; Greater palatine approach to intra-oral maxillary nerve block

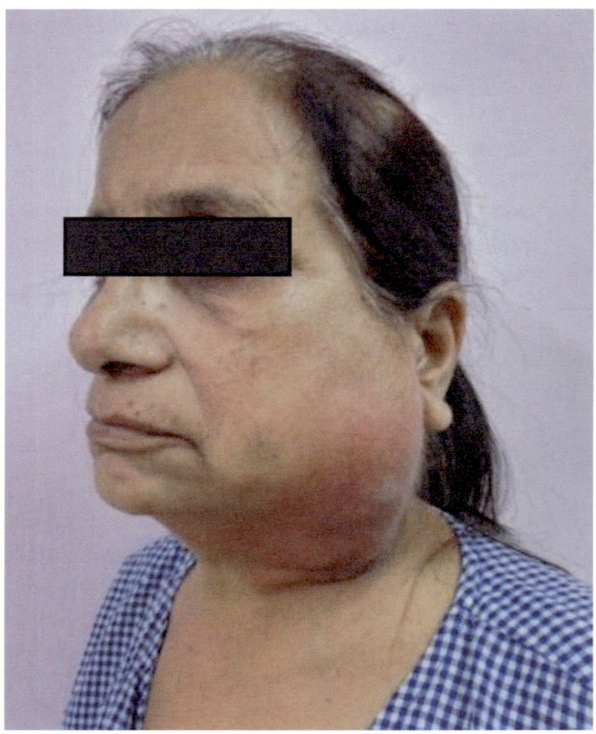

Fig. 6 Infection of fascial spaces of head and neck after repeated alcohol injection threatening the airway

Clinical Pearls

- Anatomical landmarks are important for any of the intra-oral nerve blocks.
- Application of topical anesthesia at the target area helps reducing pain caused by needle insertion.

References

1. Mckenzie KG. The surgical treatment of trigeminal neuralgia. Can Med Assoc J. 1925;15:1119–24.
2. Gregg JM, Small EW. Surgical management of trigeminal pain with radiofrequency lesions of peripheral nerves. J Oral Maxillofac Surg. 1986;44:12225.
3. Stajic Z, Juniper RP, Todorovic L. Peripheral streptomycin/lidocaine injections versus lidocaine alone in the treatment of idiopathic trigeminal neuralgia. A double blind controlled trial. J Craniomaxillofac Surg. 1990;18:243–6.
4. Chindia ML, Ng'ang'a PM. Alcohol injection in the management of paroxysmal trigeminal neuralgia: a report of 6 cases. East Afr Med J. 1994;71:49–50.
5. Handerson WR. Trigeminal neuralgia: the pain and its treatments. Brit Med. 1967;1:7–15.
6. Oturai AB, Jensen K, Erikson J, Marsden F. Neurosurgery for trigeminal neuralgia: comparison of alcohol block, neurectomy and radiofrequency coagulation. Clin J Pain. 1996;12:311–5.

Part III

Surgical Treatment of Trigeminal Neuralgia

Glycerol Rhizolysis for Trigeminal Neuralgia

Hari Hara Dash

Key Points

- Percutaneous procedures are safe and effective in treating drug-refractory trigeminal neuralgia (TGN)
- Percutaneous retrogasserian glycerol rhizolysis (PRGR) is cost-effective, easy to perform with an image intensifier, and provides immediate pain relief for a variable time-period
- Complications during and after PRGR are comparable to other percutaneous techniques

Introduction

A plethora of percutaneous procedures are available for the management of trigeminal neuralgia (TGN). Percutaneous procedures are useful in patients with drug-refractory TGN, who either refuse surgery, or in those with significant medical risks to undergo invasive surgical procedures. Percutaneous retrogasserian glycerol rhizolysis (PRGR) is one of the most popular methods of treatment for TGN. PRGR is carried out by injecting anhydrous glycerol into the Meckel's cave and its safety has been established by several studies [1–4]. The major advantages of PRGR are: (1) long-term pain relief following single injection, (2) significant reduction in

H. H. Dash (✉)
Anesthesiology and Pain Management, Fortis Memorial Research Institute (FMRI), Gurugram, Haryana, India

G. P. Rath (ed.), *Handbook of Trigeminal Neuralgia*,
https://doi.org/10.1007/978-981-13-2333-1_18

postoperative facial deafferentation compared to thermal rhizotomy, and (3) simple to perform with an image intensifier. Precise anatomic placement of anhydrous glycerol is achieved with the help of intraoperative trigeminal water-soluble contrast cisternography prior to drug injection [5–8].

Indications

PRGR may be the first-line treatment in the following patients:

- Patients with idiopathic TGN
- Patients with significant medical comorbidities where surgical procedures such as microvascular decompression (MVD) would be very risky

PRGR is used as the second-line treatment in the following patients:

- Patients who have not responded adequately to gamma knife radiosurgery (GKRS)
- TGN secondary to multiple sclerosis (MS)
- Failure of surgical procedure such as MVD

Pre-procedural Preparation

Pre-procedural examination is important to find out associated co-morbid illnesses in the patient. Routine blood examinations carried out to rule out bleeding diathesis. Anticoagulant medications must be discontinued 5–7 days prior to the procedure. PRGR may be carried out under local anesthesia (LA) or monitored anesthesia care (MAC), with or without sedation. Many pain physicians prescribe atropine or glycopyrrolate to prevent bradycardia during needle progression through the foramen ovale (FO) [3, 6, 7]. Transient cardiac arrest has been reported during placement of the needle through the FO [9]. Patients who are on anti-hypertensive drugs and beta blockers are advised to continue their medications on the day of procedure with a sip of water.

Procedure

PRGR can be carried out either inside the operating room (OR) or in the radiology suite. Proper imaging is important to delineate the anatomical landmarks during the procedure. Some pain physicians take the help of computed tomographic (CT) guidance or even, ultrasound, to localize the target. Single plane flat panel detector angiography system has also been described to delineate the exact position of the trigeminal ganglion [10]. Despite availability of sophisticated imaging modalities, fluoroscopic image intensifier system is popular because it is widely available and easy to operate.

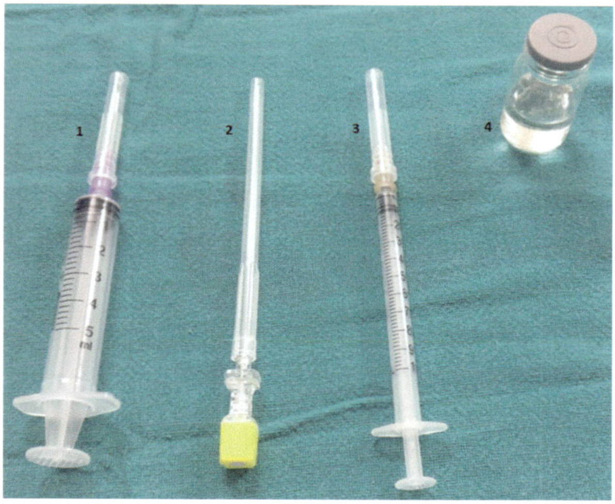

Fig. 1 Drug and equipment for retrogasserian glycerol rhizolysis; (1) 5 mL syringe, (2) spinal needle, (3) Tuberculin syringe, and (4) freshly prepared anhydrous glycerol

Drugs and Equipment (Fig. 1)

- Fluoroscopic imaging machine to identify FO and place the needle
- Disposable syringes (2 mL/5 mL)
- Local anesthetic agent (Lidocaine 2%)
- 26 G hypodermic needle
- 20/22 G spinal needle
- Freshly prepared anhydrous glycerol
- Tuberculin syringe to administer anhydrous glycerol

Technique

The procedure is performed under strict aseptic measures. The patient is placed supine with the head resting on a two-inch pillow or a head-ring, with slight extension at the atlanto-occipital joint. An intravenous (IV) cannula is secured. Continuous monitoring of electrocardiogram (ECG), heart rate, oxygen saturation and non-invasive blood pressure is obtained. Oxygen is supplemented through nasal cannula at a flow of 2–3 L/min. The image intensifier is placed to obtain a sub-mental view, and then tilted obliquely towards the affected side, until the foramen ovale (FO) is visualized, medially in relation to the mandibular process, and laterally in relation to the maxilla. The C-arm position is then adjusted in such a way that the FO is seen as an oval-shaped opening (Fig. 2a). Skin of the affected side of face is prepared with antiseptic solutions. Classic **Hartel's technique** is most commonly used to access the trigeminal cistern or the retrogasserian region via FO [3–6]. The tip of a spinal needle (22 G) may be used as metal marker and placed on the middle of the FO with the help of fluoroscopy. A skin wheal is raised 2.5–3 cm lateral to the angle of mouth with a 26 G hypodermic needle, after local

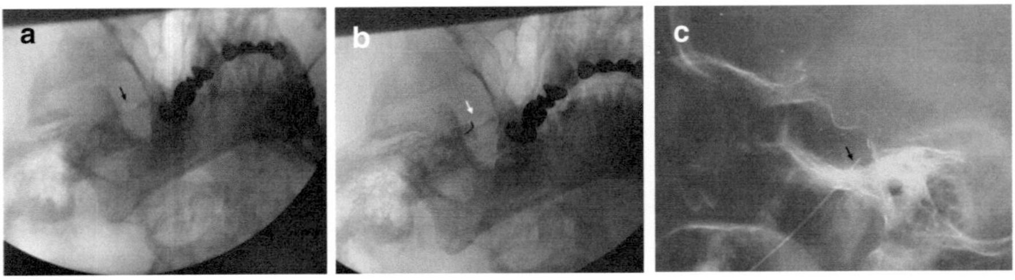

Fig. 2 Submental view shows oval-shaped foramen ovale (black arrow) (**a**), spinal needle insertion in a tunnel view (white arrow) (**b**) followed by confirmation of the position of needle tip with lateral view (black arrow) (**c**)

infiltration with 2% lidocaine. The needle is advanced through the skin wheal into the subcutaneous tissue pointing the tip of the needle towards the midpoint of the zygomatic process; 3–5 mL of 2% lidocaine is injected for adequate local anesthesia along the needle tract. Under continuous fluoroscopic guidance, the spinal needle is gradually inserted by placing a finger in the same side of the mouth to prevent inadvertent insertion into the oral cavity. The needle is directed in such a way that the tip points towards the mid-pupillary plane and the hub of the needle remains in the mid-zygomatic plane. The most painful part of the procedure is when the needle enters the FO. This may induce hypertension and at times, severe bradycardia. Close observation of hemodynamic parameters at this stage is important. Cardiac arrest has been reported during needle placement through the FO, presumably due to stimulation of trigemino-cardiac reflex. In such circumstances, the needle should be promptly withdrawn to restore cardiac activity [9]. After placement of the needle in a tunnel view (Fig. 2b), lateral view of the skull is obtained to find out the depth of the needle penetration (Fig. 2c). The tip of the needle should not cross beyond the level of the clivus.

Once the needle is in the trigeminal cistern, stylet is removed and egress of CSF is observed. If no flow is observed, the needle may be advanced further at 1 mm increments, under continuous fluoroscopic guidance, until the trigeminal cistern is entered. At times, CSF may not egress due to clogging of the needle tip with tissue, debris or blood. Some practitioners may inject a small volume of 2% lidocaine (0.25 mL) into the hub of the needle, which helps to clear the needle lumen allowing free flow of CSF. Sometimes, the egress of CSF is not observed, but the patient develops hypoesthesia on the injected side, which is a confirmatory sign of correct needle placement in the trigeminal cistern. Although CSF flow is desirable, its absence does not preclude identification of the trigeminal cistern [1, 3, 11].

Rhizolysis of Individual Divisions: Placement of the needle on the lateral and middle parts of FO blocks the mandibular division [6, 7]. If the needle is advanced through the middle part of FO and placed a little beyond the mid portion of the clivus and the foramen, it blocks the maxillary division [6, 7]. To block the ophthalmic division, the needle is placed towards the medial aspect of FO, such that the tip remains just below the clivus [6, 7].

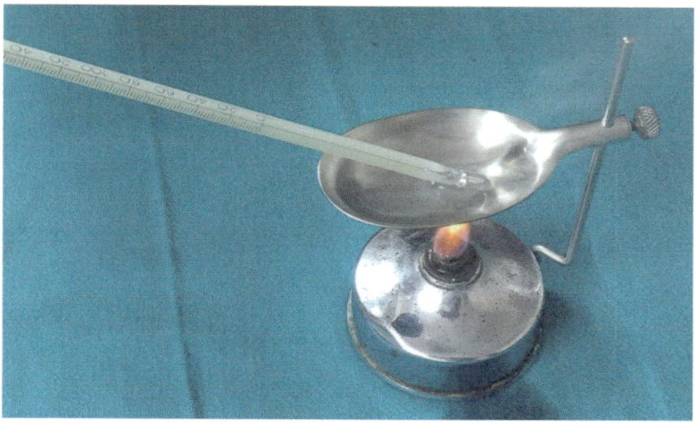

Fig. 3 Preparation of anhydrous glycerol using burner along with a thermometer to measure the temperature continuously

Preparation of Anhydrous Glycerol: Glycerol commonly available in the pharmacy is not anhydrous. To make it anhydrous, glycerol is heated at 180 °C for 45–60 min in a Bunsen burner (Fig. 3) [2]. Anhydrous glycerol can also be prepared heating the glycerol inside an electric oven at 180 °C for 1 h [2].

Administration of Glycerol: Once the tip of the needle is in the trigeminal cistern, 0.3–0.4 mL of Iohexol (Omnipaque) contrast medium is injected to obtain cisternography. Delineation of the trigeminal cistern in the shape of a pear, or a sphere, helps in further confirmation of the trigeminal ganglion [12]. The dye is aspirated and the patient is allowed to sit. Freshly prepared anhydrous glycerol 0.25–0.4 mL is taken in a tuberculin syringe and injected slowly depending on the capacity of the cisternal space (maximum capacity is 0.4–0.45 ml). There may be some discomfort in the peri-orbital region of the injected side or flushing on the injected side [3, 6, 7]. After injection of glycerol, the patient is asked to sit with the head slightly flexed for 1–2 h to prevent escape of glycerol into the posterior fossa; it allows better contact of injected glycerol with the structures in the retrogasserian area [3, 5, 8].

Mechanism of Action of Anhydrous Glycerol: Both neurolytic and osmotic effects of glycerol have been proposed [2, 5]. Glycerol is a weak alcohol, which selectively causes neuroablation of large myelinated fibres that are already damaged by the pathologic processes of TGN [13, 14]. Hakanson contended that small myelinated and unmyelinated fibres appear to be less vulnerable to the effects anhydrous glycerol than large fibres [1]. Another proposed mechanism of action is that anhydrous glycerol insulates the pathological site on the axon, and because it has a high dielectric constant (45.5 at 25 °C), it makes the nerve a poor conductor. This causes presynaptic inhibition and delays impulse propagation through the nerve [15].

Complications

- Immediate
  - Injection site hematoma
  - Inadvertent entry of needle into the oral cavity
  - Vasovagal attack, severe bradycardia and transient cardiac arrest

  - Hypertensive episodes
  - Excruciating pain while entering the foramen ovale
- Late Complications
  - Mild hypoesthesia on the injected side
  - Dysesthesia, anesthesia dolorosa
  - Corneal hypoesthesia
  - Activation of dormant Herpes simplex virus in the Gasserian ganglion
  - Motor paresis of mandibular nerve
  - Rarely, aseptic meningitis

Outcome

Udupi and colleagues retrospectively compared PRGR and radiofrequency thermocoagulation (RFT) in 79 patients with TGN [16]. It was observed that more patients in RFT group had excellent pain relief compared to PRGR group (84% vs. 58%). However, the mean duration of excellent pain relief in both groups were similar, and more patients in the RFT group had recurrence of pain compared to PRGR group (51% vs. 39%) [16]. Noorani and colleagues carried out a retrospective study comparing three percutaneous procedures—PRGR, RFT and percutaneous balloon compression (PBC) for TGN [17]. They found that PBC provided longer duration of pain relief, but with a slightly higher rate of transient side-effects [17]. In another study, the effectiveness of PRGR was assessed prospectively by studying the blink reflex, which involves the fifth and seventh cranial nerves, before and after PRGR. The authors found better function on the contralateral side following pain relief after glycerol rhizotomy [18]. In a recently published retrospective cohort study, both PBC and PRGR were found to be effective as primary surgical treatment methods in TGN, however, the side-effects were less common with PBC technique [19]. In a prospective comparative study of 45 patients undergoing either PBC or PRGR, recurrence as well as complications were significantly higher in PBC procedures compared to PRGR [20]. The authors of another prospective study of 93 patients, who were treated with PRGR, concluded that it is a simple, minimally-invasive and cost-effective method of treating drug-refractory TGN [21]. This study found immediate post-procedure pain relief in 97% patients, long-term pain control in nearly 90% patients, and only 10% recurrence rate at 18 months [21].

Conclusion

PRGR provides immediate and long-lasting pain relief in patients with drug-refractory TGN. It is a minimally-invasive, safe, relatively simple, and cost-effective procedure, with very few side effects or complications. Most of the side-effects can be prevented by proper identification of anatomic structures under continuous fluoroscopic guidance.

References

1. Hakanson S. Trigeminal neuralgia treated by the injection of glycerol in trigeminal cistern. Neurosurgery. 1981;9:38–46.
2. Saini SS. Injection treatment of trigeminal neuralgia with special reference to the use of anhydrous glycerol. Neurol India. 1981;29:31–4.
3. Lunsford LD. Treatment of tic douloureux by percutaneous retrogasserian glycerol injection. JAMA. 1982;248:449–53.
4. Arias MJ. Percutaneous retrogasserian glycerol rhizotomy for trigeminal neuralgia. J Neurosurg. 1986;65:32–6.
5. Saini SS. Reterogasserian anhydrous glycerol injection therapy in trigeminal neuralgia: observations in 552 patients. J Neurol Neurosurg Psychiatry. 1987;50:1536–8.
6. Burchiel KJ. Percutaneous retrogasserian glycerol rhizolysis in the management of trigeminal neuralgia. J Neurosurg. 1988;69:361–366.8.
7. Kondziolka D, Lunsford LD. Percutaneous retrogasserian glycerol rhizotomy for trigeminal neuralgia: technique and expectations. Neurosurg Focus. 2005;18:E7.
8. Dash HH. Management of patients with Trigeminal neuralgia. J Anaesth Clin Pharmacol. 1999;15:541–3.
9. Rath GP, Dash HH, Prabhakar H, Pandia MP. Cardiorespiratory arrest during anhydrous glycerol injection for trigeminal rhizolysis. Anaesthesia. 2007;62:971–2.
10. Arishima H, Kawajir S, Arai H, Higashino Y, Kodera T, Kikuta K. Percutaneous glycerol rhizotomy for trigeminal neuralgia using a single plane, flat panel detector angiography system: technical note. Neurol Med Chir (Tokyo). 2016;65:257–63.
11. Pandia MP, Dash HH, et al. Does egress of cerebro-spinal fluid during percutaneous retrogasserian glycerol rhizotomy influence by long term pain relief? Reg Anesth Pain Med. 2008;33:222–6.
12. Lunsford LD. Identification of Meckel cave during percutaneous glycerol rhizotomy for Tic Douloureux. AJNR. 1982;3:680–2.
13. Pal HK, Dinda AK, Roy S, Banerji AK. Acute effect of glycerol on peripheral nerve: An experimental study. Br J Neurosurg. 1989;3:463–9.
14. Normikko TJ, Eldridge PR. Trigeminal neuralgia - pathophysiology, diagnosis and current treatment. Br J Anaesth. 2001;87:117–32.
15. Calvin WH, Loeser JD, Howe JF. A neurophysiological theory for the pain mechanism of tic douloureux. Pain. 1977;3:147–54.
16. Udupi BP, Chouhan RS, Dash HH, Bithal PK, Prabhakar H. Comparative evaluation of percutaneous retrogasserian glycerol rhizolysis and radiofrequency thermocoagulation techniques in the management of trigeminal neuralgia. Neurosurgery. 2012;70:407–12.
17. Noorani I, Lodge A, Vajramani G, Sparrow O. Comparing percutaneous treatments of trigeminal neuralgia: 19 years' experience in single centre. Stereotact Funct Neurosurg. 2016;94:75–85.
18. Kumar R, Mahapatra AK, Dash HH. Blink reflex before and after percutaneous glycerol rhizolysis in patients with trigeminal neuralgia: a prospective study of 28 patients. Acta Neurochir. 1995;137:80–5.
19. Asplund P, Blomstedt P, Bergenheim AT. Percutaneous balloon compression vs percutaneous retrogasserian glycerol rhizotomy for the primary treatment of trigeminal neuralgia. Neurosurgery. 2016;78:421–8.
20. Kouzounias K, Lind G, Schechtmann G, Winter J, Linderoth B. Comparison of percutaneous balloon compression and glycerol rhizotomy for the treatment of trigeminal neuralgia. J Neurosurg. 2010;113:486–92.
21. Kodeeswaran M, Ramesh VG, Saravanan N, Udesh R. Percutaneous retrogasserian glycerol rhizotomy for trigeminal neuralgia: a simple, safe, cost-effective procedure. Neurol India. 2015;63:889–94.

Radiofrequency Thermocoagulation for Trigeminal Neuralgia

Parmod Kumar Bithal

Key Points

- Radiofrequency thermocoagulation (RFT) for trigeminal neuralgia (TGN) offers a number of benefits over other percutaneous procedures
- It is precise and gives the highest initial success rate with low incidence of recurrence
- It avoids damage to the unaffected division(s) of the trigeminal nerve, and the affected branch can be localized by application of stimulation
- Two types of radiofrequency ablation modes for Gasserian ganglion are in vogue: continuous and pulsed radiofrequency
- Common complications of RFT such as diminished corneal sensation and masseter muscle weakness usually recover over a period of time

Introduction

Trigeminal neuralgia (TGN) can be managed medically, surgically, or by percutaneous techniques. Among the percutaneous techniques, radiofrequency thermocoagulation (RFT) offers many benefits over others. The radiofrequency (RF) current is a low energy, high frequency (50–500 kHz), alternate current. When RF current is delivered to the biological tissues, it causes oscillation of the molecules within the

P. K. Bithal (✉)
Division of Neuroanesthesiology, Department of Anesthesiology and OR Administration, King Fahad Medical City, Riyadh, Kingdom of Saudi Arabia

G. P. Rath (ed.), *Handbook of Trigeminal Neuralgia*,
https://doi.org/10.1007/978-981-13-2333-1_19

tissue. That leads to production of heat by friction between the oscillating particles [1]. A lesion is formed if the temperature within the neuronal tissue exceeds 40 °C [2]. Two different modalities of RF currents are commonly practiced in interventional pain medicine: (1) Continuous radiofrequency (CRF) and (2) Pulsed radiofrequency (PRF). In CRF, an alternate current in the frequency range of 100–500 kHz is applied continuously to a target nerve; the aim is to produce a thermal lesion thereby causing interruption of afferent pathways for nociception [1]. The thermal (Heat) energy is produced transversely along the active tip of the electrode. Hence, an alignment of the active tip is usually desired alongside of the nerve targeted, and not perpendicular to it [3]. In PRF, an alternate current is applied to the target nerve without generating significant heat. Typically, high frequency current of 50 kHz is delivered over 20 ms pulses at a frequency of 2 Hz, for a duration of 120 s. The long pause between pulses results in heat dissipation, thereby keeping tissue temperature below neuro-destructive threshold of 45 °C. Pulsing the current also allows the generator power output to be substantially increased. The usual voltage output in CRF is 15–25 V, while PRF is usually carried out at 45 V. Heating is further minimized by restricting electrode tip temperature below 42 °C. Thus, the low temperature in the tissues is insufficient to produce neural lesion. In contrast to CRF, the distal active tip is desired to be perpendicular to the target nerve in PRF, as it allows delivery of highest intensity with such a placement [1].

Indications

The following patients of TGN are ideal candidates for RFT:

- Primary TGN not controlled satisfactorily with medications, or if patient is intolerant to the side effects of medications
- Patients unwilling to undergo craniotomy for microvascular decompression (MVD)
- Elderly patients, patients with limited life span, or patients at high risk for MVD
- Patients with recurrent trigeminal neurovascular compression
- Recurrence of pain following RFT

Advantages of Radiofrequency Thermocoagulation (RFT)

The technique of RFT of Gasserian ganglion (GG) for TGN was popularized by Sweet and Wepsic in 1974 [4]. The procedure requires only sedation in most of the patients and is usually carried out as a day care procedure in an operating room setup (Fig. 1). It offers the benefit of being precise, reproducible and effective. It has the advantage of stimulation before ablation to avoid damaging the wrong nerve element, thereby, providing a safety margin. In addition, it is a safe and viable

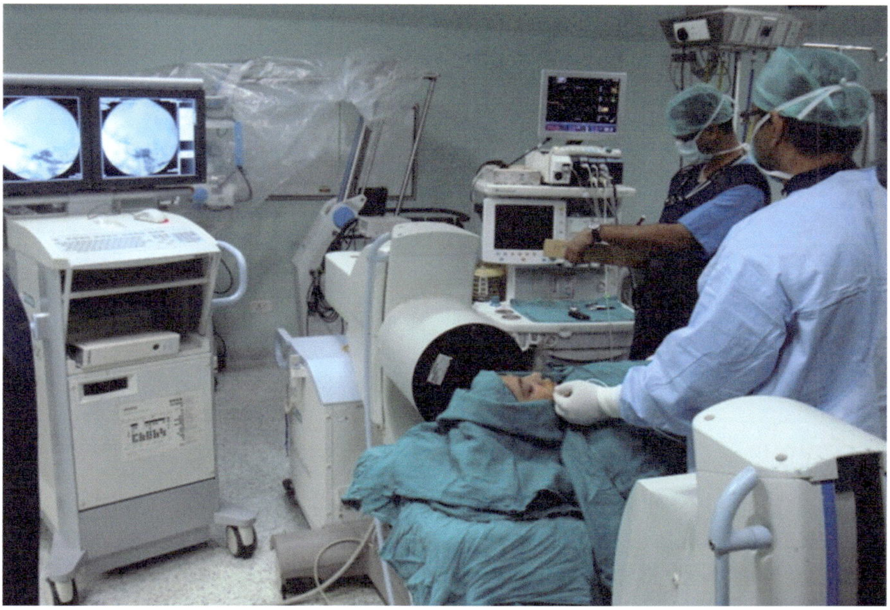

Fig. 1 Setup for radiofrequency thermocoagulation in trigeminal neuralgia

option for poor surgical risk or elderly patients, who are at high risk for MVD because morbidity and mortality are lower with RFT. Among all interventional percutaneous pain therapies, RFT offers the highest rate of complete pain relief [5]. Although 15–20% of patients may experience recurrence of pain within 12 months of the procedure; the recurrence rate is lowest among all percutaneous techniques [6]. The goal of thermocoagulation is to produce mild-to-moderate hypoalgesia in the affected division(s), thereby, allowing adequate pain relief without significant sensory deficit.

Equipments

RFT set for TGN includes the following:

- Syringe (5 mL)
- Local anesthetic (lidocaine 2%)
- Trigeminal neuralgia kit (Fig. 2) and RF generator
- Image intensifier fluoroscope (C-arm)

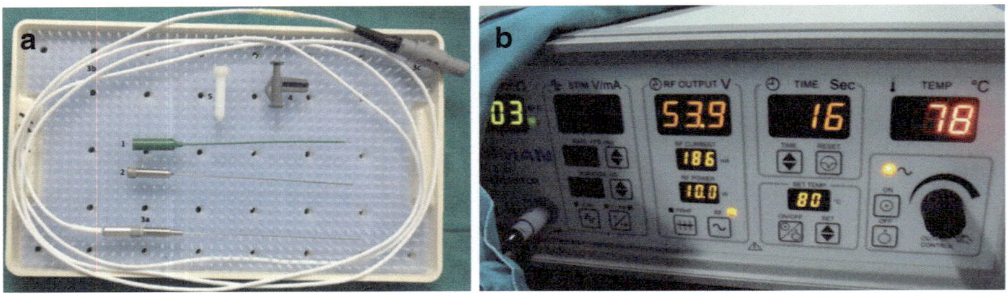

Fig. 2 Trigeminal neuralgia kit (**a**) with cannula (1), stylet (2), straight electrode (3a) attached to the cable (3b) and connector to the radiofrequency (RF) generator, flushing adapter (4), and depth stop (5); RF generator for thermocoagulation (**b**)

Technique

Standard fasting of 6–8 h is recommended in patients prior to the procedure. Sedation with propofol is usually necessary for patient comfort. To visualize the foramen ovale (FO), the fluoroscope (C-arm) is positioned in mento-orbital plane. Under all aseptic measures and after local anesthetic infiltration, a 10-cm long, 22 G cannula with 5–mm active tip is advanced from a point about 3 cm lateral to the ipsilateral angle of mouth, in a co-axial manner (tunnel view) to the X-ray beam towards the FO. When it is observed from the front, the needle trajectory appears to be toward the ipsilateral pupil, and when looked from the side, it passes 3 cm anterior to the external auditory meatus [6]. Needle insertion may also be carried out with the C-arm image intensifier in lateral position (Fig. 3a). A finger should be placed in the mouth during needle advancement to rule out breach in the buccal mucosa. When the cannula tip enters the FO, the depth is ascertained on lateral fluoroscopic view (Fig. 3b). The electrode is advanced 2–4 mm further through the canal of the foramen. Finally, the tip of the electrode is placed at the junction of petrous ridge of temporal bone and the clivus. Appropriate precaution needs to be taken to avoid placement of the electrode 10 mm beyond the clivus as trochlear and abducens nerves present there may get injured [7]. The stylet is then withdrawn from the cannula and gentle aspiration may be performed to ensure that there is no cerebrospinal fluid (CSF) or blood. Injection of 0.5 mL contrast dye helps confirm the needle has not penetrated the dura [8]. The entire procedure is guided by C-arm fluoroscopy. After placement of the needle electrode, the patient is awakened, and sensory and motor assessments are made. Test stimulation is mandatory before any RF lesioning. The mandibular nerve lies in the lateral portion of the FO. If mandibular nerve is stimulated at 0.1–0.2 V and at a frequency of 2 Hz, muscle contraction is observed at the lower jaw [9] which confirms passage of the needle through FO with the tip placed in the trigeminal roots. Paraesthesia is reproduced at 0.1–0.5 V and 50 Hz frequency in the concordant trigeminal distribution of the patient's usual symptoms [8]. If paraesthesia is obtained above 0.5 V stimulation, the needle should be redirected to achieve a similar response at a lower voltage. After appropriate stimulation parameters have been obtained, 0.5 mL of 0.5% bupivacaine should be injected. After a wait period of at least 30 s, lesions are

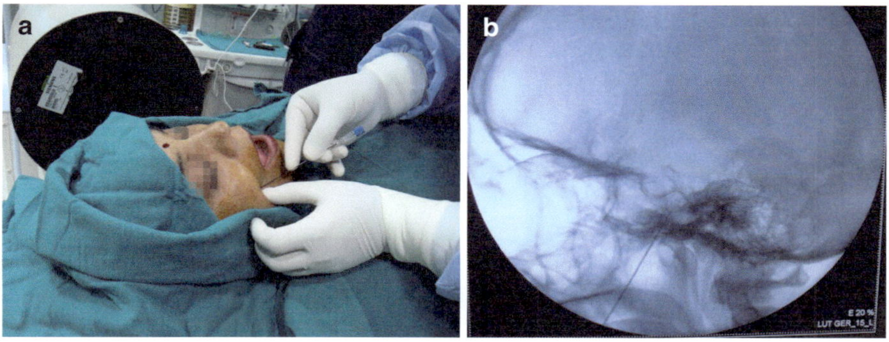

Fig. 3 Needle placement (**a**) and confirmation with lateral fluoroscopic view (**b**)

made at a maximum of 0.5 V for 30 s to 2 min. A temperature ranging from 60–90 °C is usually used for RFT of TGN [10]. To avoid discomfort, the patient should be sedated with propofol during lesioning. The needle is usually repositioned to repeat RF lesioning if more than one branch is involved. Serious complications often occur at a temperature more than 70 °C while RFT at lower temperature leads to poor pain relief [11].

Although the procedure is performed under sedation and monitored anesthesia care (MAC), general anesthesia (GA) may have to be administered in elderly patients, in whom it is challenging to transition between deep (for placement of RF needle and lesioning) and light sedation (for stimulation studies). GA may also be required in patients who are unable to tolerate, or who do not prefer to be awake during the procedure. It has been observed that pain relief is comparable when the procedure is carried out under GA, or the traditional method with sedation [12]. Patil et al. described the stereotactic method that enables the placement of the cannula, and an intraoperative computed tomographic (CT) scan that helps to confirm accurate electrode placement [13].

For the second division (maxillary nerve) and multiple divisions TGN, long-term pain relief after RFT may be less compared to isolated third division (mandibular nerve) neuralgia [14]. RFT for second or multiple divisions TGN is technically more challenging than for isolated third division neuralgia because of its anatomical distribution. Hence, the duration of pain relief in these patients appears to be shorter despite excellent immediate result. The mechanism of difference in duration of response in patients with mandibular division and with multiple divisions TGN could be the result of anatomical and/or technical difficulties of selective thermocoagulation to approach maxillary nerve fibres. When treating maxillary nerve pain, adjusting the position of the electrode is technically difficult because it requires to be positioned more medially and deeper to come in contact with the maxillary nerve fibers. If advanced too deep, it affects the ophthalmic nerve fibers, which could result in the reduction or loss of corneal sensation [15]. Nevertheless, for maxillary TGN, and combined maxillary and mandibular TGN, even if the electrode comes in contact with only the inferior portion of maxillary fibres, thermal effects of RF could spread to destroy the upper part of maxillary nerve fibres. This could be the reason for the high immediate success rate;

however, the durability of nerve destruction by diffuse heat may not last as long as that by direct effects. The probability of being pain free is considerable lower in maxillary TGN than in isolated mandibular TGN, for which direct lesion is easy to make.

Characteristics of RF Lesioning and Histological Changes

The lesion dimension depends on the size of the electrode, temperature generated, duration of radiofrequency applied, and the characteristics of local tissue. The lesion is usually oval-shaped, parallel to the needle and commonly should not exceed the tip of the needle. Hence, the needle should be placed parallel to the target nerve in ideal circumstances; a 15° curve may allow better targeting of the lesion [16]. However, there is no report till date regarding the rate of recurrence with curved tip electrode compared to straight tip electrode [17]. Following the lesioning, the tissues first develop coagulation, followed by acute inflammatory reaction, necrosis and collagen formation. This whole process takes about 3 weeks. However, since the basal lamina is often preserved and the nerve regenerates over time. RFT allows preferential destruction of pain conducting fibres such as Aδ and C-fibers while it preserves the heavily myelinated Aβ fibers that conduct touch sensation [18].

Factors Influencing Lesion Size

Tissue characteristics such as fluid contents, specifically blood or CSF, which act as heat sink, can influence the lesion size. The tissue heating decreases rapidly as the distance from the electrode tip increases. Therefore, RFT lesions are well-circumscribed and thus, advantageous as compared glycerol rhizolysis in terms of precision. Most authors recommend pulling out the cannula until there is no CSF flow.

Efficacy and Factors Predicting Pain Relief

The initial pain relief may vary following percutaneous RFT of GG; however, the success rates are generally high. Pain relief may be achieved in up to 98% of patients, which is comparable to the success rate following MVD [8]. With RFT, pre-procedure pain characteristic is the most significant predictor associated with successful outcome. Provoked paroxysmal pain has been found to be associated with higher rate of successful outcome with RFT [8]. On the other hand, bilateral TGN, high baseline numerical rating pain score, or associated psychiatric conditions, atypical and mixed type TGN, are related with less successful outcomes [19, 20]. The success of RFT is proportional to the extent of post-procedure hypoesthesia.

Studies have claimed that RFT is a useful procedure in patients of TGN secondary to multiple sclerosis. In these patients the success rate and durability of pain relief of RFT matches that of RFT in idiopathic TGN [21, 22].

Pulsed Radiofrequency

Pulsed radiofrequency (PRF) utilizes brief pulses of high frequency alternate current to produce the same voltage or even higher fluctuations than during conventional RF treatment. However, excessive heat build-up in the tissues is avoided to prevent tissue coagulation. PRF does not produce thermal lesions, but evidences suggest that microscopic damage can occur within the axonal microfilaments and microtubules; the changes are greater in C-fibers than Aβ or Aδ fibers [23]. Both RFT and PRF cause distance-dependent tissue destruction; with RFT, the effect is more pronounced. It has been suggested that the acute effects of PRF are reversible and less destructive than that of RFT.

The early published case reports on PRF showed contradictory results. Subsequently, it was realized that as compared to RFT alone, the combined effect of RFT and PRF can achieve comparable pain relief with lesser side effects [24]. Moreover, PRF can reduce complications like anesthesia dolorosa and hyperesthesia or shorten the recovery time after complications due to RFT [25]. History of MS or surgery does not influence the response rate to PRF. It has been reported that PRF at a higher voltage and larger pulse width obtains an increased rate of pain relief [26]. Overall, the results of various studies have demonstrated that PRF is not as effective as CRF thermocoagulation. To achieve better results, the PRF and RFT should be considered to be complimentary techniques rather than alternative treatment modalities [27].

Hemodynamic Effects of Radiofrequency Thermocoagulation

RFA stimulates marked pressor response resulting in rise of blood pressure and this response remains positive only below temperature of 75 °C [28]. This correlation becomes negative above 75 °C [28].

Complications

- **Corneal anesthesia and masseter weakness** (up to 20%): Common side effects are related to damage of the fifth nerve
- **Corneal complications** are more likely to occur; as compared to other percutaneous procedures. The patients recover from the complications over a period of time, however, vision may be lost if keratitis develops
- **Dysesthesia and numbness** may occur in the distribution of the treated division of the nerve
- **Anesthesia dolorosa** is extremely disturbing to the patient and difficult to treat
- **Diplopia** (less common) may occur and is caused by thermal damage to trochlear and abducens nerves [5]
- **Intracranial bleeding** can also occur. It is rare but a serious complication [29], probably due to sudden rise in blood pressure due to heating of trigeminal rootlets

- **Meningitis** may occur in 0.15% cases [30]. The effectiveness of antibiotic prophylaxis is not established, but, it should be administered when breach in the oral mucosa occurs.

Incidence of complications can be reduced by using neuronavigation, electrophysiology of GG, stereotactic approach combined with three-dimensional computed tomographic (3D CT) reconstruction models, all of which can improve accuracy in patients with difficult access to FO [31, 32].

Conclusion

The selection of percutaneous technique should be done after causes like neurovascular compression by magnetic resonance imaging (MRI) are ruled out. However, in elderly patients with multiple comorbid conditions, percutaneous procedures are selected to avoid risk of open neurosurgery. RFT is currently one of the most commonly utilized treatment options in this scenario. CRF is widely used, as the efficacy of PRF for the management of TGN is controversial.

References

1. Rea W, Kapur S, Mutagi H. Radiofrequency therapies in chronic pain. Contin Educ Anaesth Crit Care Pain. 2011;11:35–8.
2. Slappendel R, Crul B, Braak GJ, Geurts JW, Booji LH, Voerman VF, de Boo T. The efficacy of radiofrequency lesioning of the cervical spinal dorsal root ganglion in a double blind randomized study: no difference between 40 degrees C and 67 degrees C treatments. Pain. 1997;73:159–63.
3. Lord SM, Bagduk N. Radiofrequency procedures in chronic pain. Best Pract Res Clin Anesthesiol. 2002;16:597–617.
4. Sweet WH, Wepsic JG. Controlled thermocoagulation of trigeminal ganglion and rootlets for differential destruction of pain fibers. J Neurosurg. 1974;40:143–56.
5. Kanpolat Y, Savas A, Bekar A, Berk C. Percutaneous controlled radiofrequency trigeminal rhizotomy for the treatment of idiopathic. Trigeminal neuralgia: 25 years' experience with 1600 patients. Neurosurgery. 2001;48:532–4.
6. Emril DR, Ho K. Treatment of trigeminal neuralgia: role of radiofrequency ablation. J Pain Res. 2010;3:249–54.
7. Wang JY, Dender MT, Bettegowda C. Percutaneous procedures for the treatment of trigeminal neuralgia. Neurosurg Clin N Am. 2016;27:277–95.
8. Raj PP, Lou L Erdine S, Staats PS, Waldman SD, editors. Radiographic imaging for regional anesthesia and pain management. Philadelphia PA: Churchill Livingstone; 2003.
9. Koizuka S, Saito S, Kubo K, Tomioka A, Takazawa T, Sakurazawa S, Goto F. Percutaneous radiofrequency mandibular nerve rhizotomy guided by CT fluoroscopy. AJNR. 2006;27:1647–8.
10. Tang YZ, Wu BS, Yang LQ, Yue JN, He LL, Li N, et al. The long term effective rate of different branches of idiopathic trigeminal neuralgia after single radiofrequency thermocoagulation. Medicine (Baltimore). 2015;94:e1994.

11. Nie F, Su D, Shi Y, Chen J, Wang H, Chen Y, et al. A prospective study of x-ray imaging combined with skin stimulation potential- guided percutaneous continuous radiofrequency thermocoagulation of the Gasserian ganglion for the treatment of trigeminal neuralgia. Pain Med. 2014;15:1464–9.
12. Hart MG, Nowell M, Coakham HB. Radiofrequency thermocoagulation for trigeminal neuralgia without intraoperative patient waking. Br J Neurosurg. 2012;392:110–5.
13. Patil AA, Chamczuk AJ, Nelson B. Stereotactic radiofrequency ablation of trigeminal ganglion with intraoperative CT scan and under general anesthesia. Open J Modern Neurosurg. 2016;6:55–9.
14. Kosugi S, Shiotani M, Otsuka Y, Suzuki T, Kotari N, Hashguchi S, Morisaki H. Long term outcomes of percutaneous radiofrequency thermocoagulation of Gasserian ganglion for 2nd and multiple-division trigeminal neuralgia. Pain Pract. 2015;15:223–8.
15. Fraioli B, Epsosito V, Guidetti B, Cruccu G, Manfredi M. Treatment of trigeminal neuralgia by thermocoagulation, glycerolization and percutaneous compression of the Gasserian ganglion and/or retrogasserian rootlets: long term results and therapeutic protocols. Neurosurgery. 1989;24:239–45.
16. Finch PM. A curved approach to nerve blocks and radiofrequency lesioning. Pain Digest. 1997;7:251–7.
17. Tobler WD, Tew JM Jr, Cosman E, Keller JT, Quallen B. Improved outcome in the treatment of trigeminal neuralgia by percutaneous stereotactic rhizotomy with a new, curved tip electrode. Neurosurgery. 1983;12:313–7.
18. Laghmari M, El Ouahahi A, Arkha Y, Derraz S, El Khamlichi A. Are the destructive neurosurgical techniques as effective as microvascular decompression in the management of trigeminal neuralgia. Surg Neurol. 2007;68:505–12.
19. Jin HS, Shin JY, Kim YC, Lee SC, Choi EJ, Lee PB, Moon JY. Predictive factors associated with success and failure for radiofrequency thermocoagulation in patients with trigeminal neuralgia. Pain Physician. 2015;18:537–45.
20. Yizhong H, Jiaxiang NI, Baishan WU, Mingwei HE, Liqiang Y, Wang Q. Percutaneous radiofrequency thermocoagulation for the treatment of different types of trigeminal neuralgias: evaluation of quality of life and outcomes. J Huazhong Univ Sci Technolog Med Sci. 2010;30:403–7.
21. Sindou M, Tatli M. Treatment of trigeminal neuralgia with thermocoagulation. Neurochirurgia. 2009;55:203–10.
22. Bender MT, Pradilla G, Batra S, See AP, James C, Prado CA, et al. Glycerol rhizotomy and radiofrequency thermocoagulation for trigeminal neuralgia in multiple sclerosis. J Neurosurg. 2013;118:329–36.
23. Bogduk N. Pulsed radiofrequency. Pain Med. 2006;7:396–407.
24. Li X, Ni J, Yang L, Wu B, He M, Zhang X, Ma L, Sun H. A prospective study of Gasserian ganglion pulsed radiofrequency with continuous radiofrequency for the treatment of trigeminal neuralgia. J Clin Neurosci. 2012;19:824–8.
25. Zhao WX, Wang Q, He MW, Yang B, Wu S, Ni JX. Radiofrequency thermocoagulation combined with pulsed radiofrequency helps relieve postoperative complications of trigeminal neuralgia. Genet Mol Res. 2015;14:7616–23.
26. Luo F, Meng L, Wang T, Yu X, Shen Y, Ji N. Pulsed radiofrequency treatment for idiopathic trigeminal neuralgia: a retrospective analysis of the causes for ineffective pain relief. Eur J Pain. 2013;17:1189–92.
27. Liao C, Visocchi M, Liu P, Zhang W. Pulsed radiofrequency: a management option for recurrent trigeminal neuralgia following radiofrequency thermocoagulation. World Neurosurg. 2017;97:760.e5–7.
28. Meng Q, Zhang W, Yang Y, Zhou M, Li X. Cardiovascular responses during percutaneous radiofrequency thermocoagulation therapy in primary trigeminal neuralgia. J Neurosurg Anesthesiol. 2008;20:131–5.

29. Rath G, Dash HH, Bithal PK, Goyal V. Intracranial hemorrhage after percutaneous trigeminal rhizotomy. Pain Pract. 2009;9:82–4.
30. Ward L, Khan M, Greig M, Dolin SJ. Meningitis after percutaneous radiofrequency trigeminal ganglion lesion. Case report and review of literature. Pain Med. 2007;8:535–8.
31. Yang Y, Shao Y, Wang H, Liu Y, Zhu S, Wu C. Neuronavigation assisted percutaneous thermocoagulation in trigeminal neuralgia. Clin J Pain. 2007;23:159–64.
32. Guo Z, Wu B, Du C, Cheng H, Tian Y. Stereotactic approach combined with 3D CT reconstruction for difficult to access foramen ovale on radiofrequency thermocoagulation of the Gasserian ganglion for trigeminal neuralgia. Pain Med. 2016;17:1704–16.

Percutaneous Microballoon Compression for Trigeminal Neuralgia

Virender Kumar Mohan and Debesh Bhoi

Key Points

- Percutaneous Gasserian ganglion (GG) microballon compression (PMBC) is considered as an effective modality for treatment of trigeminal neuralgia (TGN)
- Large myelinated fibers are damaged with compression leaving the unmyelinated fibers intact and thus, corneal reflex is preserved
- Pear-shaped appearance of microballon after inflation with the dye indicates accurate positioning of the tip, and hence, a good clinical outcome is predicted
- Significant hemodynamic changes occur in the initial phase of compression leading to bradycardia; hence, atropine-filled syringe may be kept attached to an intravenous access for prompt treatment

Introduction

In patients of trigeminal neuralgia, (TGN) early surgical intervention is indicated, when medical therapy becomes refractory (Level C) [1]. Microvascular decompression (MVD) is the standard surgical option, when there is a neurovascular compression in the Meckle's cave. However, elderly patients with multiple

V. K. Mohan (✉) · D. Bhoi
Department of Anaesthesiology, Critical Care, and Pain Medicine, All India Institute of Medical Sciences (AIIMS), New Delhi, India

G. P. Rath (ed.), *Handbook of Trigeminal Neuralgia*,
https://doi.org/10.1007/978-981-13-2333-1_20

co-morbid conditions are not suitable candidates for such complex posterior fossa surgeries [2, 3].

Percutaneous microballoon compression (PMBC) of Gasserian ganglion (GG) and gamma knife radiosurgery (GKRS) are considered as next modalities (Level C). PMBC was first described in 1983 by Mullan and Lichtor [4]. They showed compression of the nerve led to more significant and long-lasting effects than the decompression. Mullan improvised this technique and compressed the GG with 4F Fogarty embolectomy balloon catheter to relieve pain [5]. In PMBC, the trigeminal root is compressed by the microballoon of Fogarty catheter, introduced through a wide bored (14G) needle under fluoroscopic guidance. Inflation of the balloon leads to damage the large myelinated fibers which are responsible for sensory trigger for the trigeminal pain. The unmyelinated fibers are preserved; hence, the corneal reflex remains intact. Thus, PMBC provides immediate pain relief with advantage of being safe and simple.

Patient Selection

Before planning for PMBC, a high-resolution brain stem, trigeminal, and vessel imaging is done to look for any neurovascular compression (NVC), that might be managed with MVD. However, in cases of failed MVD, multiple sclerosis, idiopathic TGN without NVC, involvement of multiple divisions, or in patients with multiple co-morbid diseases, the PMBC is considered as a viable alternative [6]. Atypical facial pain, post-herpetic neuralgia, and contralateral masseter weakness are few relative contraindications for PMBC.

Preparations

PMBC is a day-care procedure performed under general anesthesia (GA). Each patient is thoroughly evaluated for the presence of co-morbidities, difficult airway, or anesthesia-related issues. Investigations such as complete hemogram, renal function tests, coagulation profile, and 12-lead electrocardiography (ECG) are carried out. Written informed consent is obtained from each patient after the possible outcome and procedure-related complications are explained. Standard fasting guidelines are followed night prior to the procedure. In the operation theatre (OR), an intravenous (IV) access is secured and routine monitoring modalities such as continuous ECG, non-invasive blood pressure (NIBP), pulse oximetry (SpO_2), and $EtCO_2$ are connected. An atropine-filled syringe is always attached to the IV line for prompt treatment significant bradycardia which may occur as a complication of the procedure. Transcutaneous pacing pads may also be attached for the same purpose.

Equipments

The following agents and equipment are required for percutaneous trigeminal ganglion compression (Fig. 1).

- Metal marker
- 14 G/13 cm needle
- 23 G/10 cm spinal needle for deeper local anesthetic injection
- A micro balloon catheter (4F Fogarty catheter)
- Syringes (5 and 2 mL)
- 1 ml insulin syringe filled with Iohexol dye non-ionic radio contrast material

Technique

The patient is placed supine, head is slightly extended, a roll is placed below the shoulder, and face is turned to the opposite side. Skin of the face and anterior neck is prepared with topical antiseptics, and is draped with sterile towels. A sub-mental view (slight lateral and oblique) is obtained using C-arm image intensifier to visualize foramen ovale (FO). Foramen ovale is a small, translucent circular/oval shaped image just medial to mandibular arch, above the petrous bone. A metal marker used to mark the skin entry which is approximately 2–2.5 cm lateral and 0.5 cm cephalad to angle of mouth [4]. Other important landmarks are middle of the pupil and a point 2.5–3 cm anterior to external auditory meatus or middle of the zygoma (Fig. 2). Needle with sharp stylet is inserted towards the mid-pupil if seen from above and towards the middle of zygoma if seen from the side. Once the needle is engaged to FO, the direction and depth is to be checked fluoroscopically with a lateral view (Fig. 3). The tip of the needle should be in line with the point where clivus joins the petrous part of temporal bone just below the entry of FO. Another approach is starting needle insertion in sub-mental view (Fig. 4). The needle is inserted in a tunnel view and advanced parallel to C-arm image intensifier beam in a co-axial manner to reach the entry of FO. During initial placement of the needle, one finger is placed inside the mouth to avoid penetration of oral mucosa which is a possible risk factor for the occurrence of post-procedural meningitis. Once the needle is engaged into the FO, the direction and depth would be checked fluoroscopically in lateral view. After the needle position is ascertained, the stylet is withdrawn; and the needle hub should be looked for any backflow of CSF or blood. There might be slight bleeding from the epidural veins but not from an artery. A pre-marked 4F fogarty catheter (1 cm mark beyond the length of needle) is then introduced, approximately 1.4–1.7 cm beyond the tip in order to place the balloon in the Meckel's cave. The guidewire of forgarty catheter is removed, and cuff is inflated slowly with 0.7–1.0 mL of radio-opaque contrast material (iohexol) with a tuberculin syringe or an insufflator

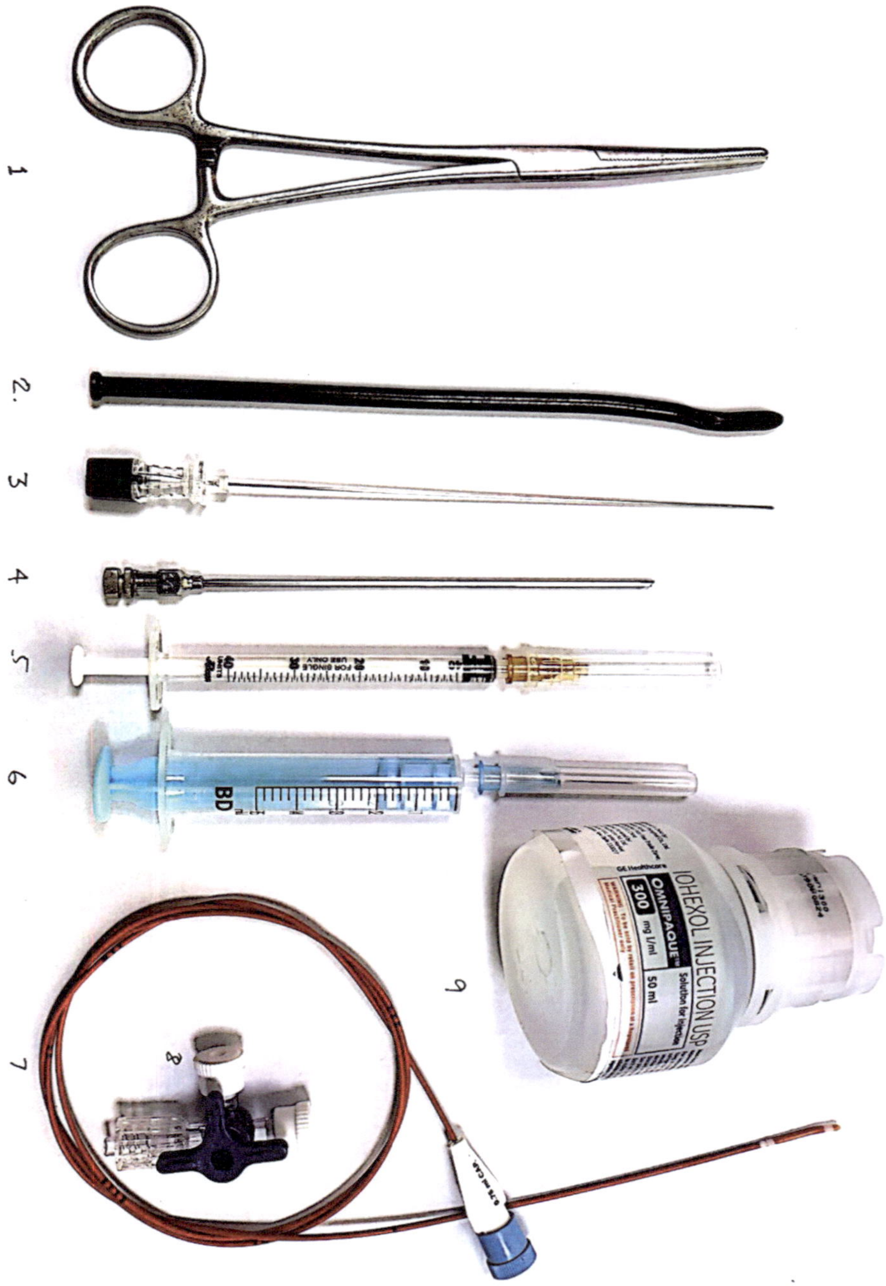

Fig. 1 Instruments used during procedure: (1) Artery forceps; (2) Metal markers; (3) Spinal needle; (4) Procedure needle; (5/6) Syringes with hypodermic needles; (7) Fogarty embolectomy catheter; (8) 3-way stopcock; (9) Radio-contrast material

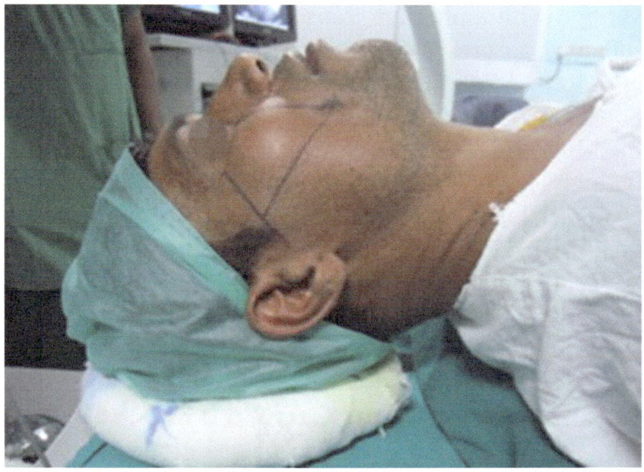

Fig. 2 Patient position and skin marking used during needle insertion

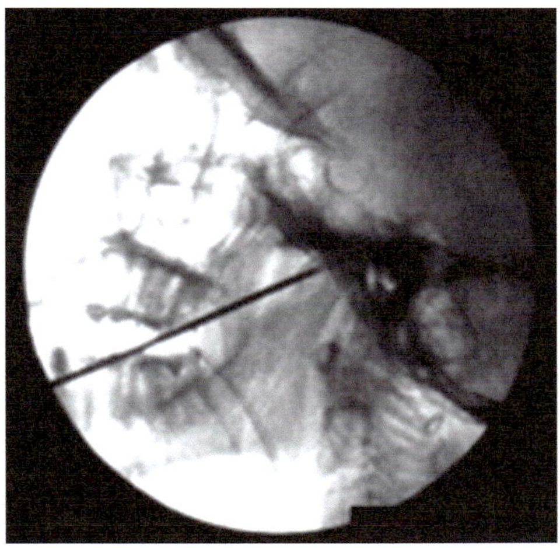

Fig. 3 Fluoroscopic lateral view showing needle tip at the entrance of foramen ovale (FO) in line with the point where clivus meets the petrous part of the temporal bone

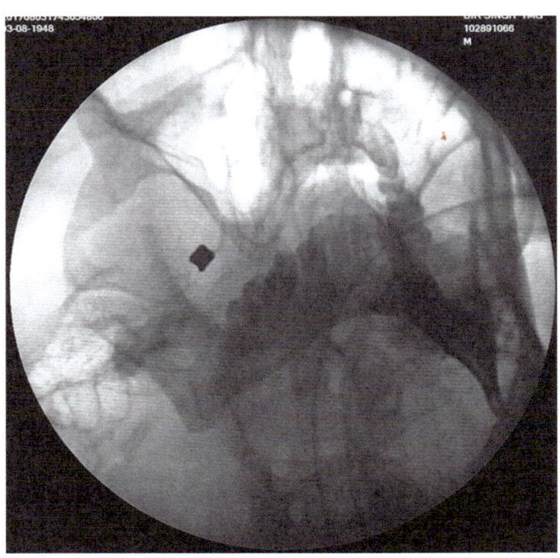

Fig. 4 Fluoroscopic sub-mental view showing the needle entering the foramen ovale (FO)

syringe with a pressure transducer under continuous fluroscopic guidance. Before inflation, air present should be aspirated to stabilize the intraluminal pressure. With appropriate inflation, a pressure of 1200–1500 mmHg can be achieved [7]. The appearance of pear-shaped balloon, indicates that it is beginning to protrude out of the Meckel's cave towards posterior fossa; and a good squeeze can be achieved. The balloon is kept inflated for 60 s or more and then deflated under continuous fluoroscopic vision after which the assembly are withdrawn as a single unit. CSF leak may occur if the catheter is withdrawn, separately. The catheter should be checked for any tear, and entry site is compressed for 5 min with sterile gauze piece, and aseptic dressing follows.

Mechanical Changes Caused by PMBC

There occur few anatomic changes inside the Meckel's cave after PMBC which depend upon the location, volume, and size of the microballoon [8]. Significant changes occur when the forgarty catheter tip is located on the porus trigemini which is 15–20 mm beyond the FO. At this site, the fully distended balloon (volume 0.75–1.0 mL) assumes a pear shape.

Neural Effects: A neural compression is produced between the balloon surface and the inner dural wall, at the level of GG causing dispersion and spreading of the nerve fibers, both motor as well as sensory.

Dural Effects: Elevation and stretching of the gasserian dura occurs as a consequence of balloon inflation. The area of stretching is initially small but eventually reaches an average surface area of 15×10 mm^2, distally to the porus trigemini and medially to the lateral wall of the cavernous sinus. On withdrawal of the balloon, the dura of cavum turns flaccid.

Shape of the Balloon

The different balloon shapes observed are pear, dumb-bell, round, elliptical, or irregular [9]. When accurately positioned, it assumes a "***pear shape***" with its stem end facing posteriorly (Fig. 5). It is formed when the tip of the fully inflated balloon is inserted into the slenderer area of the porus trigemini, posteriorly to the ganglion, beyond which it may slip into the posterior fossa adjacent to brain stem [5]. The petrous bone restricts it inferiorly and the firm surrounding of dural edge superiorly, where the sensory root is compressed [3]. Because of the varying size of the cave, the ideal shape is not always possible to achieve.

The balloon shape is an important predictor of the outcome following PMBC. Mullan and Lichtor suggested continued inflation of the balloon until the pear-shape is achieved which correlated with a good result and minimal numbness [4]. Elliptical shape is associated with poor pain relief and recurrences representing an infratemporal lateral position of the balloon. This position could be adjusted with the help of a frontal fluoroscopic view [10].

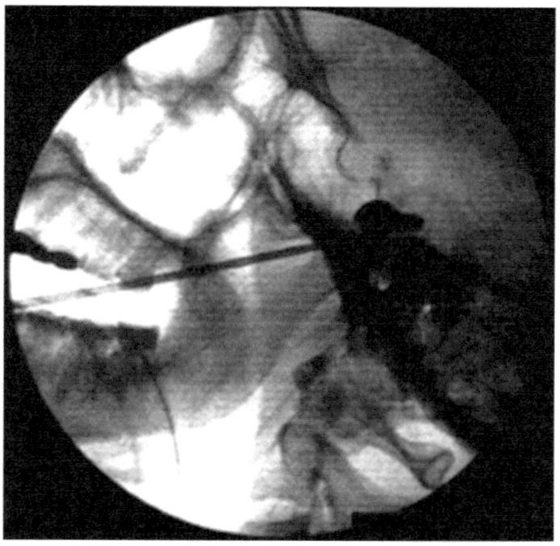

Fig. 5 Fluoroscopic lateral view showing catheter in place and pear-shaped inflated balloon

The intraluminal balloon pressure is another crucial factor affecting outcome thereby limiting the therapeutic effect if it is below 600 mmHg [11]. The pressure exerted is in direct relationship with and depends on the resistance to stretching by the dura.

Stylet/Catheter Adjustments during the Procedure (for division specific compressions): In an antero-posterior view, the center of petrous bone is brought to the orbit area, where a dip on the bone is observed; it is the proximal entrance for the porous trigeminus. Stylet/balloon is placed in the middle of porous for V2 or multi-division compressions, at the lateral aspect for V3, and medially, for the compression of V1 division. The porous trigeminus is located within 17–20 mm from the FO, hence, the catheter-tip should not be placed further. For V3, the tip should be placed 2 mm further to the edge of petrous bone, and slight further for the V1 division.

Trigemino-Cardiac Reflex (TCR): There occur significant hemodynamic changes during PMBC and the most salient one is sudden bradycardia, observed during initial phase of ganglion compression [4, 12]. Continuous intraoperative hemodynamic monitoring should be done to avoid bradycardia leading to asystole [13, 14] and syringe filed atropine should also be kept attached to an IV access. Both sympathetic and parasympathetic systems are involved in TCR. Administration of labetalol prior to ganglion compression has also been found to decrease the severity of bradycardia [15–17].

Complications

The common complications associated with PMBC are dysesthesia, masseter weakness and paralysis, diminished/absence of corneal sensation, anesthesia dolorosa, cranial nerve injury, and aseptic meningitis. Other rare complications include carotid cavernous fistula [18], sub-arachnoid hemorrhage [19], and aneurysm formation [20]. Cranial nerve damage has been reported in 0–3% cases, after percutaneous interventional procedures for TGN [21]. The damage involves optic, oculomotor, trochlear, abducens, facial, and vestibulo-cochlear nerves [22, 23]. The abducens nerve is the most commonly affected cranial nerve [22] as it enters the cavernous sinus at lower edge of the inferomedial **paraclival triangle**. The triangle is formed by line extending from the posterior-clinoid process to the dural entrance of the trochlear nerve as its base. Lateral border of the triangle is formed by a line joining dural entrance of the trochlear to abducens nerves whereas the line connecting the dural entrance of abducens nerve to the posterior-clinoid process forms the medial border. Balloon compression of lateral wall of the cavernous sinus causes mechanical damage with resultant sixth nerve palsy [22]. Ocular nerve palsies are uncommon after PMBC [24].

Masseter weakness is a common complication, and expected in all patients receiving PMBC. It is possibly due to focal demyelination of the motor branch after PMBC. It may take 6–12 months for the muscle function to recover from such weakness [23].

Sudden reversible blindness has been reported in a patient after a PMBC of GG [25], which could be due to sudden increase in intraocular pressure as a result of occlusion of venous drainage of the orbit. It was reversed with appropriate medical treatment.

Transient diplopia occured in four patients out of 144 patients in a series of case underwent PMBC [11]. Mullan and Lichtor observed trochlear nerve palsy in one patient as a consequence of dural arterio-venous malformation (AVF), that lasted for 3 months [4]. Isolated reversible trochlear nerve palsy has been observed in a patient after PMBC [26]. It occurs due to compression of the fourth cranial nerve, at its entry to the cavernous sinus, by the protruded part (through the porus trigemini) of inflated microballoon into the posterior fossa. It can be prevented by appropriate placement of Fogarty catheter, careful inflation of the balloon, and avoidance of further penetration into the posterior fossa [26].

Successful Compression

There is no specific consensus regarding the compression time or compression pressure. A better outcome is achieved with a longer compression time [27]. A higher pressure and prolonged compression time are associated with increased chance of complications such as numbness, dysthesia, and masseter weaknesses [28]. Lichtor and Mullan noticed decreased incidence of dysthesia when the compression time was reduced from 6–7 min to 1 min.

Recurrence

Incidence of immediate pain relief after PMBC ranges from 80% to 90% [29–31]; patients usually remain without medication for 2–3 years. The recurrence rate varies from 10% to 30%. It depends on factors like TGN owing to multiple sclerosis or inability to attain a pear-shape during balloon compression. Occurrence of numbness along the distribution of pain predicts good outcome with analgesia with a lesser chance of recurrence [9]. The rate is low where PMBC is done at the earliest then in those with long-gap between appearance of the symptom and the procedure [32].

Conclusion

PMBC is a simple and effective procedure with better compliance which is usually performed under light general anesthesia. It is associated with minimal complications; and a successful procedure improves the quality of life in patients suffering from trigeminal neuralgia.

References

1. Cruccu G, Gronseth G, Alksne J, Argoff C, Brainin M, Burchiel K, Nurmikko T, Zakrzewska JM, American Academy of Neurology Society, European Federation of Neurological Society. AAN-EFNS guidelines on trigeminal neuralgia management. Eur J Neurol. 2008;15:1013–28.
2. Brown JA. Percutaneous balloon compression for trigeminal neuralgia. Clin Neurosurg. 2009;56:73–8.
3. Revuelta-Gutierrez R, Martinez-Anda JJ, Coll JB, Campos-Romo A, Perez-Peña N. Efficacy and safety of root compression of trigeminal nerve for trigeminal neuralgia without evidence of vascular compression. World Neurosurg. 2013;80:385–9.
4. Mullan S, Lichtor T. Percutaneous microcompression of the trigeminal ganglion for trigeminal neuralgia. J Neurosurg. 1983;59:1007–12.
5. Shelden CH, Pudenz RH, Freshwater DB, Crue BL. Compression rather than decompression for trigeminal neuralgia. J Neurosurg. 1955;12:123–6.
6. Yadav YR, Yadav N, Pande S, Parihar V, Ratre S, Khare Y. Trigeminal neuralgia. Asian J Neurosurg. 2017;12:585–97.
7. Gerber AM. Improved visualization of the foramen ovale for percutaneous approaches to the gasserian ganglion. Technical note. J Neurosurg. 1994;80:156–9.
8. Urculo E, Martinez L, Arrazola M, Ramirez R. Macroscopic effects of percutaneous trigeminal ganglion compression (Mullan's technique): an anatomic study. Neurosurgery. 1995;36:776–9.
9. Kouzounias K, Schechtmann G, Lind G, Winter J, Linderoth B. Factors that influence outcome of percutaneous balloon compression in the treatment of trigeminal neuralgia. Neurosurgery. 2010;67:925–34.
10. Park SS, Lee MK, Kim JW, Jung JY, Kim IS, Ghang CG. Percutaneous balloon compression of trigeminal ganglion for the treatment of idiopathic trigeminal neuralgia: experience in 50 patients. J Korean Neurosurg Soc. 2008;43:186–9.
11. Lobata RD, Rivas JJ, Sarabia R, Lamas E. Percutaneous microcompression of the gasserian ganglion for trigeminal neuralgia. J Neurosurg. 1990;72:546–53.
12. Brown JA, Preul MC. Trigeminal depressor response during percutaneous microcompression of the trigeminal ganglion for trigeminal neuralgia. Neuro-surgery. 1988;23:745e8.
13. Belber CJ, Rak RA. Balloon compression rhizolysis in the surgical management of trigeminal neuralgia. Neurosurgery. 1987;20:908e13.
14. Arasho B, Sandu N, Spiriev T, Prabhakar H, Schaller B. Management of the trige-minocardiac reflex: facts and own experience. Neurol India. 2009;57:375e80.
15. Dominguez J, Lobato RD, Rivas JJ, Gargallo MC, Castells V, Gozalo A, Sarabia R. Changes in systemic blood pressure and cardiac rhythm induced by therapeutic compression of the trigeminal ganglion. Neurosurgery. 1994;34:422e7.

16. Bereiter DA, Gann DS. Adrenal secretion of catecholamines evoked by chemical stimulation of trigeminal nucleus caudalis in the cat. Neuroscience. 1988;25:697e704.
17. Chen CY, Luo CF, Hsu YC, Chen JF, Day YJ. Comparison of the effects of atropine and labetalol on trigeminocardiac reflex-induced hemodynamic alterations during percutaneous microballoon compression of the trigeminal ganglion. Acta Anaesthesiol Taiwan. 2012;50:153–8.
18. Langford P, Holt ME, Danks RA. Cavernous sinus fistula following percutaneous balloon compression of the trigeminal ganglion. Case report. J Neurosurg. 2005;103:176–8.
19. Spaziante R, Cappabianca P, Peca C. Subarachnoid hemorrhage and normal pressure hydrocephalus-fatal complication of percutaneous microcompression of the Gasserian ganglion. Case report. Neurosurgery. 1988;22:148–51.
20. Tubbs RS, Dixon J, Loukas M, Cohen-Gadol AA. Regional vascular relationships to the foramen ovale: an anatomical study with application to approaches to the external skull base with an emphasis on transcutaneous procedures foe the treatment of trigeminal neuralgia. J Neurosurg. 2010;113:493–7.
21. Lopez BC, Hamlyn PJ, Zakrzewska JM. Systemic review of ablative neurosurgical techniques for the treatment of trigeminal neuralgia. Neurosurgery. 2004;54:973–82.
22. Kefalopoulou Z, Markaki E, Constantoyannis C. Avoiding abducens nerve palsy during the percutaneous balloon compression procedure. Stereotact Funct Neurosurg. 2009;87:101–4.
23. Chroni E, Constantoyannis C, Prasoulis I, Kargiotis O, Kagadis GC, Georgiopoulos M, Polychronopoulos P. Masseter muscle function after percutaneous balloon compression of trigeminal ganglion for the treatment of trigeminal neuralgia: a neurophysiological follow-up study. Clin Neurophysiol. 2011;122:410–3.
24. Ahn KS, Lee MK, Hwang SH, Lee JE, Cho CW, Kim DJ. Percutaneous balloon compression of trigeminal ganglion for the treatment of idiopathic trigeminal neuralgia. J Korean Neurosurg Soc. 2004;36:213–7.
25. Agazzi S, Chang S, Drucker MD, Youssef AS, Van Loveren HR. Sudden blindness as a complication of percutaneous trigeminal procedures: mechanism analysis and prevention. J Neurosurg. 2009;110:638–41.
26. Urculo E, Alfaro R, Arrazola M, Astudillo E, Rejas G. Trochlear nerve palsy after repeated percutaneous balloon compression for recurrent trigeminal neuralgia: Case report and pathogenic considerations. Neurosurgery. 2004;54:505–8.
27. Li F, Han S, Ma Y, Yi F, Xu X, Liu Y. Optimal duration of percutaneous microballoon compression for treatment of trigeminal nerve injury. Neural Regen Res. 2014;9:179–89.
28. Zanusso M, Curri D, Landi A, Colombo F, Volpin L, Cervellini P. Pressure monitoring inside Meckel's cave during percutaneous micro-compression of gasserian ganglion. Stereotact Funct Neurosurg. 1991;56:37–43.
29. Bergenheim AT, Asplund P, Linderoth B. Percutaneous retrogasserian balloon compression for trigeminal neuralgia: review of critical technical details and outcomes. World Neurosurg. 2013;79:359–68.
30. Brown JA, McDaniel MD, Weaver MT. Percutaneous trigeminal nerve compression for treatment of trigeminal neuralgia: results in 50 patients. Neurosurgery. 1993;32:570–3.
31. Tatli M, Satici O, Kanpolat Y, Sindou M. Various surgical modalities for trigeminal neuralgia: literature study of respective long-term outcomes. Acta Neurochir. 2008;150:243–55.
32. Stomal-Słowińska M, Słowiński J, Lee TK, Uitti RJ, Deen HG, Reimer R, Cheshire WP Jr, Herzog-Bryan G, Wharen RE Jr. Correlation of clinical findings and results of percutaneous balloon compression for patients with trigeminal neuralgia. Clin Neurol Neurosurg. 2011;113:14–21.

Neurosurgical Treatment for Trigeminal Neuralgia

Sachin A. Borkar, Mohit Agrawal, and Sumit Sinha

Key Points

- Pharmacological treatment is the first line of management in trigeminal neuralgia (TGN); invasive measures preferred in drug-resistant cases
- Microvascular decompression (MVD) is the surgical treatment of choice with best outcome, in patients who are fit enough to undergo the procedure
- Other surgical modalities can be used for patients with recurrence of pain after MVD, or in patients who are unfit to undergo a major neurosurgical procedure

Introduction

Surgical procedure is warranted in trigeminal neuralgia (TGN) when pharmacologic therapy fails with insufficient pain relief or unacceptable side effects. Surgical management may broadly be divided into (a) procedures on the trigeminal nerve or gasserian ganglion by external or percutaneous approach, usually performed by pain physicians; (b) procedures carried out on the nerve root entry zone by open and invasive surgery (e.g., microvascular decompression) performed by neurosurgeons;

S. A. Borkar (✉) · M. Agrawal
Department of Neurosurgery, All India Institute of Medical Sciences (AIIMS), New Delhi, India

S. Sinha
Neurosurgery and Spine, Paras Hospital, Gurugram, India

G. P. Rath (ed.), *Handbook of Trigeminal Neuralgia*,
https://doi.org/10.1007/978-981-13-2333-1_21

Table 1 Surgical procedures for trigeminal neuralgia

Ablative procedures	Non-ablative procedures
• Retrogasserian Neurotomy • Trigeminal Tractotomy (TR) • Peripheral Neurectomy	• Microvascular decompression (MVD) • Trigeminal Internal Neurolysis (TIN)

and (c) non-invasive gamma knife (GK) radiosurgery performed by radiation oncologists and neurosurgeons. Microvascular decompression (MVD), although more invasive, has an overall superior success rate. Percutaneous techniques may be more agreeable to elderly patients who are at high surgical risk. The percutaneous procedures and GK surgery are discussed in separate chapters. This chapter elaborates open surgical procedures which may be divided into ablative/destructive procedures (e.g., peripheral neurectomy), or non-ablative procedures where the nerve function remains preserved (Table 1).

Retrogasserian Neurotomy

This was one of the earliest procedures developed for surgical treatment of TGN. It involves sectioning the trigeminal root between the gasserian ganglion (GG) and the pons. This operation is still indicated when no compression of the trigeminal nerve is discovered during suboccipital craniotomy or if MVD fails to provide long-term pain relief. Performing a partial rhizotomy lessens the probability of inducing anesthesia dolorosa and reduces the morbidity of a totally numb face. In 1934, while performing this procedure, Dandy hypothesized for the first time that the neurovascular compression may be the cause of TGN [1].

Trigeminal Tractotomy

This procedure, first descibed by Olof Sjöqvist [2] in 1938, involves destruction of the descending trigeminal tracts in the medulla. Sectioning of the descending trigeminal tract in the medulla produces isolated loss of pain and temperature sensation in the ipsilateral face and pharynx. The operation is indicated when rhizotomy has failed to alleviate pain and when all other measures have failed. It is carried out via a suboccipital craniectomy and laminectomy of C1 and C2. Computed tomographic (CT) guided procedures can be performed under local anesthesia with constant feedback from the awake patient. The largest series of CT-guided tractotomy-nucleotomy procedures have been reported by Kanpolat et al. [3] and Raslan [4]. This procedure is used for selected cases of cancer and de-afferentiation pain, atypical facial and trigeminal pain, chronic cluster headache, and vagoglossopharyngeal and geniculate neuralgias located not only in the area of the fifth, but also other nerves such as the seventh, ninth, and tenth cranial nerves. In the series by Kanpolat et al. [3], approximately 75% patients with atypical facial pain had complete pain relief over a mean follow-up period of 5.3 years. Complications included transient ataxia because of the injury to spinocerebellar tracts, Horner's syndrome due to injury to the sympathetic fibers, injury to vagus and accessory nerve nuclei, and contralateral hemiparesis.

Peripheral Neurectomy

Neurectomy is the excision of a peripheral branch of the nerve external to the skull for the relief of the neuralgia. Either an extraoral or intraoral approach can be done to access the inferior alveolar nerve (V3), infraorbital nerve (V2) or the supra orbital nerve (V1), respectively.

Peripheral neurectomy is indicated only when gangliolysis has failed and the patient might not tolerate a suboccipital craniectomy with MVD. It produces dense numbness and rarely provides more than a year of pain relief, due to nerve regeneration or growth of collaterals. Repeat avulsions of peripheral branches of the trigeminal nerve are even less likely to succeed. Pain relief can be lasting from 15 to 24 months [5]. In the series by Haiasos et al. [6] 78.7% patients had immediate pain relief with pain free duration of 30.2 months. It is a simple and safe procedure and can be performed again in case of a recurrence.

Microvascular Decompression (MVD)

The procedure is based on the rationale given by Dandy that chronic compression by blood vessels (either artery or vein or both) is the most common cause of TGN [1]. The vascular compression is found in about 96% of cases of typical TGN [7]. In the brainstem, the oligodendroglia is responsible for myelination whereas outside the brain stem, in the peripheral nervous system, the Schwann cells are responsible for myelination. This transition zone, which is named the **Redlich–Obersteiner's zone**, has a changeover from oligodendrocytes myelin to Schwann cell myelin. In this area, multiple axons have marginal or no myelination at all, thus leaving it at risk of focal de-myelination from chronic vascular compression of the trigeminal nerve. This leads to hyperactivity of the nucleus of the trigeminal nerve and resultant TGN attacks after even minimal stimulation of trigger points, such as during washing, eating, brushing teeth, or even by touching the face. The vessels most often implicated for TGN are the superior cerebellar artery (SCA), anterior and posterior inferior cerebellar arteries (AICA and PICA), and the superior petrosal vein including several of its tributaries (Fig. 1).

MVD was popularized by Jannetta [8], and hence, it is also known as **Jannetta's procedure**. The procedure is performed under general anesthesia, with the patient in lateral or supine position, with head turned to opposite side. A suboccipital retromastoid craniotomy is done after two finger-breadths incision behind ear, dura is opened to expose the cerebellum and then, the brainstem. Following which a microscope is used to visualize the trigeminal nerve as it leaves the pons. The goal of the operation is to remove the suspected compression of the nerve by the loop of blood

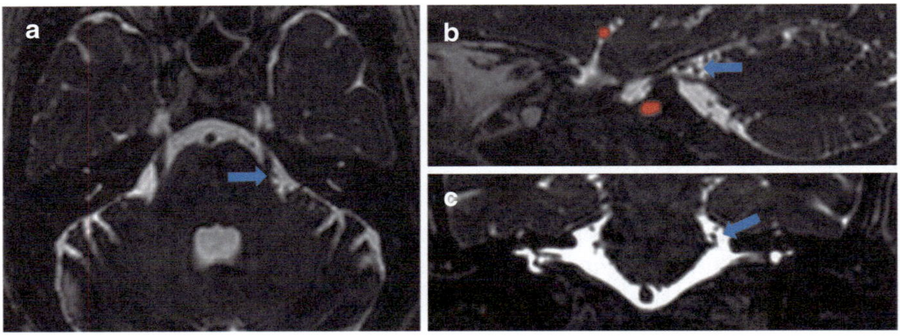

Fig. 1 Preoperative reconstructed FIESTA (heavily weighted T2) MRI images of a 32-year-old male patient with left trigeminal neuralgia. A loop of superior cerebellar artery is seen compressing at the root entry zone of left trigeminal nerve, while the right side has no abnormal loop (**a**) axial, (**b**) sagittal, and (**c**) coronal sections

vessel (either artery or vein). The offending vessel is mobilized and positioned in a new place, and partitioned from trigeminal nerve by an inert and sponge-like material, teflon. This is followed by dural closure, bone flap is replaced, and the overlying tissues are sutured in multiple layers.

Complications during MVD include cerebrospinal fluid leak (7%), transient diplopia, cranial venous thrombosis, hearing loss, facial paresis, wound infection and stroke [9]. The morbidity rate is about 5% and the mortality rate is 0.5%.

Outcome after MVD: This operation offers long term success rate and does not lead to any sensory loss. It has the best long-term success rate of any of the available surgical treatments. Acute pain relief occurs in 76.4–98.2% patients (average 91.05%), follow-up pain-free rates 62–89% (average 76.6%), and with a recurrence rate 4–38% (average 18.3%) [10]. Frail, elderly patients may not be the best candidates for this operation because of inherent risks of a major neurosurgical procedure. Factors attributing to good prognosis after MVD include typical trigeminal pain, evidence of definite vascular compression on imaging, short duration of symptoms, and no history of a former failed procedure.

- **Comparison with Gamma Knife (GK) Therapy:** MVD has an initial success rate of 89–100% as compared to 57–77% with gamma knife therapy [11–15]. Both procedures have been shown to have recurrence but MVD has a 5-year success rate of 61–80% versus 33–56% for GK [11–15]. MVD is slightly costlier as compared to GK [16], however, long-term pain relief as afforded by MVD offsets any cost advantage of GK therapy. GK is more frequently associated with complications such as numbness and dyesthetic pain as compared to MVD [11–15], which on account of being an invasive procedure is associated with some much more serious, but rare complications as described earlier. In fact, numbness is found to be an independent predictor of the pain relief outcome after GK [12, 13]. MVD has traditionally been avoided in the elderly population based on the few early reports of greater complication rate of

MVD in this patient population; on the contrary, recent studies suggest otherwise [17]. In absence of general risks of surgery and anesthesia, MVD is equally safe for the elderly patients. Another subgroup where GK is preferred is patients with no demonstrable vascular compression. However, the success rate of MVD has been observed to be greater than that of GK even in this subgroup; of course, this rate is less than those with demonstrable vascular compression [18].

- **Comparison with Partial Sensory Rhizotomy (PSR):** Gao and colleagues [19] compared the response rate between MVD and PSR at 2 weeks after surgery and it was found to be 98.08% and 84.62%, respectively. The three years recurrence rate was significantly lower in the MVD group, while the complication rate, including the occurrence of herpes was significantly higher in the PSR group.
- **Comparison with Percutaneous Balloon Compression (PBC):** Tatli et al. [10] in their review article compared the surgical outcomes of different surgical modalities and found MVD to be associated with similar rates of acute as well as follow-up pain-free rates as PBC. Acute pain relief rate was in between 97% and 100% (average 98.5%), the average follow-up pain-free rate was 80.4%. MVD was associated with the lowest rate of recurrence. MVD patients were younger than the patients undergoing PBC. Although the hospital stay was shorter in PBC group, the overall improvement of symptoms was better with MVD [20].
- **Comparison with Pharmacological Treatment:** Patients who underwent MVD were compared with carbamazepine (CBZ) and gabapentin (GBP) and analgesic block of trigger-points with ropivacaine (ROP) (GBP+ROP protocol). The GBP+ROP protocol was found to be the least expensive treatment, whereas surgery was most expensive. However, when adjusted for the time required for treatment, it was realized that the GBP+ROP protocol was most-expensive whereas MVD was least expensive technique. Therefore, in case of failure of pharmacologic approach, MVD remains the surgical method of choice [21].

Trigeminal Internal Neurolysis (TIN)

In this procedure, all or portions of the trigeminal nerve are divided longitudinally along its fibers between the pons and the porus trigeminus. This procedure is used as an alternative technique when the neurovascular compression is not observed on preoperative imaging or during surgery (MVD). Ko et al. [22] reported immediate relief of pain in 85% of patients, significant pain relief in 96% patients, with approximately 72% of patients maintaining significant pain relief without medications after 5 years. These results are comparable to those for MVD.

Endoscopic Microvascular Decompression (E-MVD)

Endoscopic technique can be used alone in TGN or as an adjuvant to microscopy. It is a minimally invasive technique [23] allows better visualization of the anatomy from the brainstem to the ganglion, including ventral aspect. This helps provide a thorough decompression of the nerve. Bohman and colleagues [24] in a series of 47 patients demonstrated excellent pain relief at a mean follow up of 15 months. None of the surgical procedure in this series was either aborted or converted to microscopic technique.

Conclusion

Proper selection of patients is essential for the surgical management of TGN. Open surgical procedures like MVD provides highest rate of patient satisfaction. In recent years there is an increasing trend for MVD in patients eligible for open surgery. Patients with typical TGN have better long-term outcomes after MVD and usually with less frequent recurrences. There is a need of large randomized controlled trials using standardized diagnostic criteria, procedures, and endpoints with respect to efficacy and safety of various procedures so that an accurate assessment of risk-benefit analysis can be made.

References

1. Dandy WE. Concerning the cause of trigeminal neuralgia. Am J Surg. 1934;24:447–55.
2. Sjöqvist O. Studies on pain conduction in the trigeminal nerve: a contribution to the surgical treatment of facial pain. Acta Psychiatr Neurol Scand Suppl. 1938;17:1–139.
3. Kanpolat Y, Kahilogullari G, Ugur HC, Elhan AH. Computed tomography-guided percutaneous trigeminal tractotomy-nucleotomy. Neurosurgery. 2008;63(1 Suppl 1):ONS147–55.
4. Raslan AM. Percutaneous computed tomography-guided radiofrequency ablation of upper spinal cord pain pathways for cancer-related pain. Neurosurgery. 2008;62(3 Suppl 1):226–34.
5. Ali FM, Prasant M, Pai D, Aher VA, Kar S, Safiya T. Peripheral neurectomies: a treatment option for trigeminal neuralgia in rural practice. J Neurosci Rural Pract. 2012;3:152–7.
6. Haliasos N, Prezerakos G, Kuruvath S, Garvan N, Bavetta S. Peripheral neurectomy as a second line treatment option for trigeminal neuralgia: 27 years' experience of a "Sidelined" procedure. Neurosurgery. 2010;67:551.
7. Meaney JF, Eldridge PR, Dunn LT, Nixon TE, Whitehouse GH, Miles JB. Demonstration of neurovascular compression in trigeminal neuralgia with magnetic resonance imaging. Comparison with surgical findings in 52 consecutive operative cases. J Neurosurg. 1995;83:799–805.
8. Jannetta PJ. Microsurgical approach to the trigeminal nerve for tic douloureux. Prog Neurosurg. 1976;7:180–200.
9. Sarsam Z, Garcia-Finana M, Nurmikko TJ, Varma TR, Eldrige P. The long-term outcome of microvascular decompression for trigeminal neuralgia. Br J Neurosurg. 2010;24:18–25.
10. Tatli M, Satici O, Kanpolat Y, Sindou M. Various surgical modalities for trigeminal neuralgia: literature study of respective long-term outcomes. Acta Neurochir. 2008;150:243–55.
11. Pollock BE. Comparison of posterior fossa exploration and stereotactic radiosurgery in patients with previously nonsurgically treated idiopathic trigeminal neuralgia. Neurosurg Focus. 2005;18:1–4.
12. Brisman R. Microvascular decompression vs. gamma knife radiosurgery for typical trigeminal neuralgia: preliminary findings. Stereotact Funct Neurosurg. 2007;85:94–8.
13. Linskey ME, Ratanatharathorn V, Peñagaricano J. A prospective cohort study of microvascular decompression and gamma knife surgery in patients with trigeminal neuralgia. J Neurosurg. 2008;109(Suppl):160–72.

14. Pollock BE, Schoeberl KA. Prospective comparison of posterior fossa exploration and stereotactic radiosurgery dorsal root entry zone target as primary surgery for patients with idiopathic trigeminal neuralgia. Neurosurgery. 2010;67:633–8.
15. Wang DD, Raygor KP, Cage TA, Ward MM, Wesycotts SS, Barbaro NM, Chang EF. Prospective comparison of long-term pain relief rates after first-time microvascular decompression and stereotactic radiosurgery for trigeminal neuralgia. J Neurosurg. 2018;128:68–77.
16. Sivakanthan S, Van Gompel JJ, Alikhani P, van Loveren H, Chen R, Agazzi S. Surgical management of trigeminal neuralgia: use and cost-effectiveness from an analysis of the Medicare Claims Database. Neurosurgery. 2014;75:220–6.
17. Sekula RF, Frederickson AM, Jannetta PJ, Quigley MR, Aziz KM, Arnone GD. Microvascular decompression for elderly patients with trigeminal neuralgia: a prospective study and systematic review with meta-analysis. J Neurosurg. 2011;114:172–9.
18. Miller JP, Magill ST, Acar F, Burchiel KJ. Predictors of long-term success after microvascular decompression for trigeminal neuralgia. J Neurosurg. 2009;110:620–6.
19. Gao J, Fu Y, Guo SK, Li B, Xu ZX. Efficacy and prognostic value of partial sensory rhizotomy and microvascular decompression for primary trigeminal neuralgia: a comparative study. Med Sci Monit. 2017;23:2284–91.
20. Jellish WS, Benedict W, Owen K, Anderson D, Fluder E, Shea JF. Perioperative and long-term operative outcomes after surgery for trigeminal neuralgia: microvascular decompression vs percutaneous balloon ablation. Head Face Med. 2008;4:1.
21. Lemos L, Alegria C, Oliveira J, Machado A, Oliveira P, Almeida A. Pharmacological versus microvascular decompression approaches for the treatment of trigeminal neuralgia: clinical outcomes and direct costs. J Pain Res. 2011;4:233–44.
22. Ko AL, Ozpinar A, Lee A, Raslan AM, McCartney S, Burchiel KJ. Long-term efficacy and safety of internal neurolysis for trigeminal neuralgia without neurovascular compression. J Neurosurg. 2015;122:1048–57.
23. Yadav YR, Parihar V, Agarwal M, Sherekar S, Bhatele P. Endoscopic vascular decompression of the trigeminal nerve. Minim Invasive Neurosurg. 2011;54:110–4.
24. Bohman LE, Pierce J, Stephen JH, Sandhu S, Lee JY. Fully endoscopic microvascular decompression for trigeminal neuralgia: technique review and early outcomes. Neurosurg Focus. 2014;37:E18.

Gamma Knife Radiosurgery for Trigeminal Neuralgia

Kanwaljeet Garg and Varidh Katiyar

Key Points

- Gamma knife radiosurgery is a non-invasive alternative to surgical procedures for the management of trigeminal neuralgia (TGN)
- It is preferred in elderly patients of TGN with medical comorbidities or patients with TGN due to multiple sclerosis
- The median latency for the onset of pain relief is about 2 months
- Sensory disturbance in the distribution of trigeminal nerve is the commonest side effect and it is dose-dependent

Introduction

Trigeminal neuralgia (TGN) is a debilitating pain syndrome. Various theories have been postulated to explain the origin of TGN [1–3]. The first-line of management includes medications such as carbamazepine, oxycarbamazepine, phenytoin, gabapentin, pregabalin, and baclofen. It is quite common that the patients become resistant to these drugs over period of time. That is the reason why many patients would require some other management strategies. The alternative treatment modalities include different surgical options which can be divided as ablative or non-ablative procedures. Microvascular decompression (MVD) is the only

K. Garg (✉) · V. Katiyar
Department of Neurosurgery and Gamma Knife, All India Institute of Medical Sciences (AIIMS), New Delhi, India

G. P. Rath (ed.), *Handbook of Trigeminal Neuralgia*,
https://doi.org/10.1007/978-981-13-2333-1_22

non-ablative surgical procedure available. The ablative procedures lead to pain relief by lesioning of the trigeminal nerve; and include percutaneous techniques such as balloon compression, retrogasserian glycerol rhizotomy, and radiofrequency lesioning. Gamma Knife radiosurgery (GKRS) is a minimal invasive technique used to control TGN.

History

Leksell used an ortho-voltage stereotactic technique to treat patients with TGN and achieved some relief of symptoms long before the development of Gamma knife (GK) [4, 5]. Since its inception by Dr. Leksell in 1971 [6] and with some early studies, the role of GKRS in patients with intractable TGN has been expanded considerably. Plain radiographs were used to visualize the gasserian ganglion in earlier days. GK did not gain much popularity in TGN early on because it was difficult to visualize the trigeminal nerve without magnetic resonance imaging (MRI). Moreover, new drugs which were introduced to control the neuropathic pain were quite effective. However, the scenario changed after the introduction of MRI.

Radiosurgery Technique

The GKRS procedure starts with the application of a Leksell stereotactic head frame (Leksell Stereotactic System®, Elekta, Stockholm, Sweden) under local anesthesia (Fig. 1). The patient then undergoes MRI; computed tomographic (CT) scan or CT cisternogram may be done in patients who cannot undergo MRI.

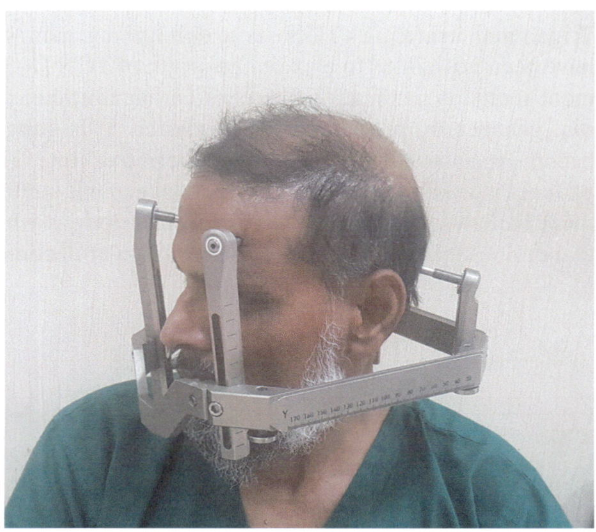

Fig. 1 A patient with Leksell head frame

Treatment Planning

In GK the collimator diameter options available are 4, 8, and 16 mm. A single shot of 4-mm beam collimator diameter is used in TGN. A single isocenter is used as the target which is very small. The isocenter is placed on the trigeminal nerve in such a way that 20% iso-dose line just touches the brainstem (Fig. 2). The final step is delivery of the radiation by the GK machine (Fig. 3).

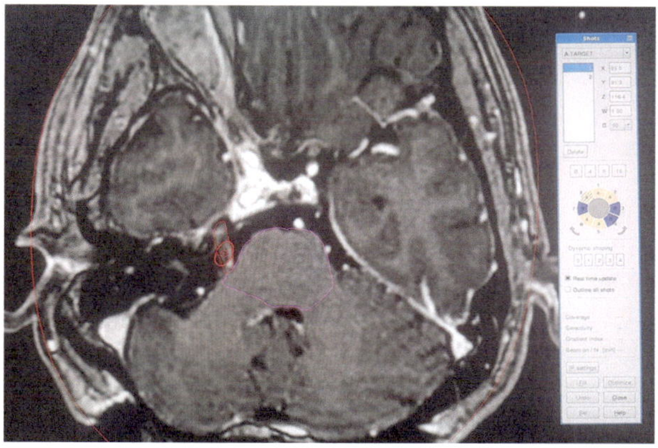

Fig. 2 Dose plan for Gamma knife in a patient with trigeminal neuralgia

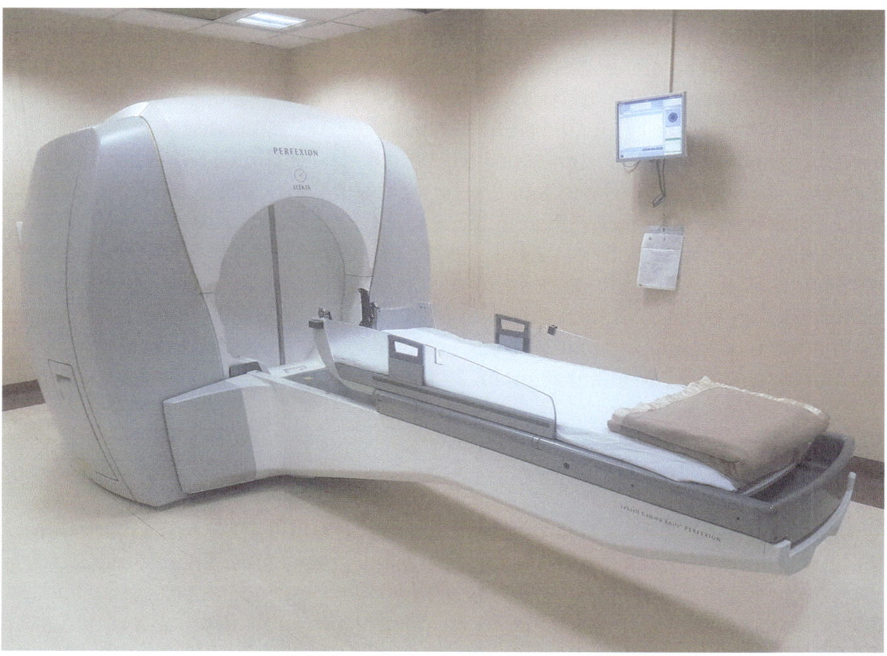

Fig. 3 Leksell Gamma knife unit (Model Perfexion)

Dose

Maximum dose used at different centres varies from 70 to 85 Gy. Reports suggest that the results are better with higher dosages, both in terms of rate of improvement and recurrence. Maximum dose has been limited to 90 Gy as higher doses can lead to serious post-radiation complications [7]. Isocenter is placed anteriorly away from the brainstem when higher dose is used. It has been demonstrated that pain control is better if 20 mm^3 of brainstem receives $\geq 20\%$ of the maximum radiation dose, than with smaller doses targeting smaller volumes [8]. Isocenter can be aligned to the trigeminal nerve by making the gamma angle to 110° [5].

Target Selection

Although the use of GKRS for TGN is now widespread, there is a lot of controversy with regard to target selection. Different target options may be close proximity to either the root entry zone (REZ) or to the gasserian ganglion, slight anteriorly. The pain relief has been suggested to be better when the GK isocenter is placed closer to the brainstem [9]. Due to the difference in the myelination pattern, the dorsal REZ has been described as a potential target for the radiation effect [10]. Analysis pertaining to initial pain control suggests that patients with the posterior target are more likely to have an excellent result [11]. The complications are significantly higher in the anterior target group. Régis et al. targeted the cisternal (distal) portion of the trigeminal root and reported excellent outcome in 87% patients with 10% having painful relapse [12]. The more anterior was the choice of target the lesser was the rate of complications, even with a maximal dose of 90 Gy. However, targeting the trigeminal nerve 5–8 mm away from the brainstem has been recommended in order to get an optimal response without significant trigeminal dysfunction [13]. The time to a response after the GK has been found to be significantly shorter in the retrogasserian zone group (mean 4.1 weeks) than in the dorsal REZ group (mean 6.4 weeks) [14].

Another variable which can have significant bearing on the GKRS planning is the length of the cisternal segment of trigeminal nerve. The dose exposed to the brainstem can be in safe limits despite high dose given to the target with longer length of the cisternal segment whereas beam shaping is required to preserve brainstem in case of short cisternal segment.

Indications

The advantage of GKRS is lack of major side effects while delay in the onset of pain relief and higher rate of recurrence are the major drawbacks. Therefore, GKRS is preferred over MVD in elderly patients who are poor candidates for general anaesthesia or those unwilling to undergo an open neurosurgical procedure [15, 16]. GKRS is also preferred in whom vascular aetiology cannot be identified like in multiple sclerosis, and the ones who have failed MVD.

Outcome

The pain relief rate in a large population of type I TGN patients 1 year after radiosurgery ranged from 75% to 90% of patients (Barrow Neurological Institute (BNI) grades I to IIIB) [9, 17–19]. Outcomes in different series of patient population are described in Table 1. TGN adversely affects quality of life (QOL), and hence, outcome of GKRS in TGN must be discussed in terms of QOL. In one study, patients with even partial pain relief reported median 80% improvement in QOL while patients with complete pain relief reported 100% improvement in QOL. The patients who had pain recurrence after pain relief reported a median 80% improvement in QOL [20].

Delay in Response

There is a median latency of 2 months before the onset of pain relief after GKRS [10, 21, 22]. Many patients who achieve partial pain relief initially can have further improvement; 1 year time period may be the optimal time to judge the effectiveness of GKRS. Kondzhiolka et al. [19] found that total pain relief was achieved at a median of 5 months. Pain relief is predicted to be faster when GKRS is performed as initial procedure, within 3 years of pain onset [19].

Persistence of Pain Relief

Good control of pain (BNI I-IIIb) is seen in 46–65% of type 1 TGN patients by 5 years after GK. Lucas et al. developed a nomogram to assess predictors of long-term pain relief after GKRS which included the type of pain at presentation, post-GK BNI score, and the presence of post-GK facial numbness [18]. Post-GK numbness was identified as a major predictor of achievement and maintenance of pain relief [9, 19, 23]. Patients showing an early response within the first three weeks may also experience a longer duration of complete pain relief [24].

Prognostic Factors

The factors which have been found to have good correlation with favourable outcome are younger patient age, length of trigeminal nerve irradiated, neurovascular conflict on MRI, higher dose of radiation, and proximity of isocenters to brainstem [23, 25]. Poor prognostic factors include atypical facial pain and presence of multiple sclerosis [21, 26]. Results of GKRS in TGN are better if it is used as an initial treatment modality than as secondary treatment modality [21, 26].

Table 1 Results of gamma knife radiosurgery in patients with trigeminal neuralgia: literature review

Studies	No. of patients	Median follow-up (months)	Mean age	Dose (Gy) mean (range)	Time to pain response (days)	Prior surgery (%)	Good facial pain outcome (%)	Treatment failure	Recurrence
McNatt et al. (2005)	49	23 (5–55)	68	80 (80–80)	37.5	21	61	39	23
Sheehan et al. (2005)	136	11 (6–22)	68	80 (50–90)	24 (1–180)	54	90 1 year 70 3 years	10	24
Régis et al. (2006)	100	19 (2–96)	68	85 (70–90)	10 (0–175)	42	83	17	34
Fountas et al. (2007)	106	12 (36+)	72	80/85 (75–85)	28	46	90	10	§
Longhi et al. (2007)	160	12 (1–60)	63	85 (75–95)	45	43	90	10	18
Dhople et al. (2009)	112	67	64	75 (70–80)	14 (0–84)	33	81	19	56
Kondziolka et al. (2010)	503	24 (3–156)	72	80 (60–90)	30 (1–365)	43	80 1 year 71 3 years	11	43
Verheul et al. (2010)	365	28 (3–85)	65	80	20 (1–150)	46	75 1 year 60 3 years	10	NA
Marshall et al. (2012)	448	21 (3–86)	67	90 (90–97)	NA	NA	86	14	40
Young et al. (2013)	250	69	70.8	90	51	11.6	89.5	6	14.3
Baschnagel et al. (2014)	149	27	70	80 (99%) 70 (1%)	21 (5–210)	34	92	8	32
Karam et al. (2013)	36	69 (36–246)	71	80–90	48 (1–180)	11	80.6	19	60
Régis et al. (2015)	497	43.8 (12–174.4)	68.3	85 (70–90)	10 (1–180)	34.8	91.8	8.25	34.4
Moreno et al. (2016)	117	66 (24–171)	64.33	86.5 (80–90)	100 (1–798)	31..62	94	6	31.82
Taich et al. (2016)	263	24 (6–48)	69	87.4 (80–97)	75	13	79	21	29.8
Chang et al. (2018)	130	106.6 (48–168)	63	78.7 (60–90)	NA	NA	81	19	7

Recurrence and Retreatment

Recurrence rate of TGN following GKRS varies from 5% to 42% and is believed to be due to incomplete effects of radiation on the targeted tissue [5]. Redo-GK is a viable treatment option owing to a favourable safety profile of GKRS. It has been shown that the response to first treatment can be used to predict response to repeat GK [21]. Results of repeat GKRS match the results of first time GK, though many patients are not able to discontinue their pain medications. New onset or worsening of facial numbness is the most common complication of repeat GKRS.

MVD vs. GKRS

MVD is considered gold standard treatment for TGN as the long-term results are very good. Maesawa and colleagues observed 70% complete pain relief at 9 months and 5 years following GKRS [21]. Whereas 27% patients were completely pain free, at last follow up, in another series [23]. Many prospective studies and a recent meta-analyses suggested MVD provides more favourable outcome than GKRS, for the treatment of TGN [27].

GKRS in TGN with Multiple Sclerosis (MS)

The incidence of TGN in MS patients is approximately 20 times of that in general population and it is frequently bilateral [28]. MS patients are less likely to tolerate neuropathic analgesics, and response is poorer as compared to non-MS patients with TGN. Response to MVD is also poor as the pathology is not vascular compression in most of the cases [28]. GKRS is a good option in these patients [28, 29]. Pain control in TGN following GKRS has been reported to be 82.6%, 73.9%, and 54.0% of patients after 1, 3, and 5 years [28]. In another series of 43 patients the probability of patients remaining pain free without medication at 6 months, 1, 3, 5 and 10 years were to be 87.2%, 71.8%, 43.1%, 38.3% and 20.5%, respectively [29]. GKRS is also associated with very low rate complications like facial sensory dysfunction which is common following percutaneous procedures [28].

Complications

The commonest side effect after GKRS is numbness or paraesthesia in trigeminal region with a reported incidence 6–66%. Matsuda et al. reported trigeminal nerve dysfunction of 49% at 3 months, which was reduced to 41.3% at a median time of 37 months [30]. Most of the patients often do not find the post-GK numbness to be troublesome [17]. Factors associated with greater risk of developing numbness include a more anterior target location, longer length of irradiated nerve, and dose utilization higher than 90 Gy [31]. In one study, the frequency of bothersome facial numbness was found to be lower in the retrogassrian group, though it was not statistically significant [14]. Other complications of GKRS include radiation-induced parenchymal changes, radiation-induced neoplasia, and vascular injury [5].

Conclusion

GKRS has become an integral part of TGN management. It is now considered an alternative to MVD for the patients with medically refractory TGN. The current recommended dose of GKRS is 80 Gy, and it achieves a pain relief rate of 60–90%. Early GKRS is associated with better outcomes in terms of pain relief, latency, as well as persistence to the response.

References

1. Dandy WE. Concerning the cause of trigeminal neuralgia. Am J Surg. 1934;24:447–55.
2. Liu Y, Li J, Butzkueven H, Duan Y, Zhang M, Shu N, et al. Microstructural abnormalities in the trigeminal nerves of patients with trigeminal neuralgia revealed by multiple diffusion metrics. Eur J Radiol. 2013;82:783–6.
3. Love S, Coakham HB. Trigeminal neuralgia: pathology and pathogenesis. Brain J Neurol. 2001;124:2347–60.
4. Leksell L. Brain fragments in radiosurgery. In: Radiosurgery: baseline and trends. New York: Raven Press; 1992. p. 623–92.
5. Zhiyuan X, Sheehan JP. Stereotactic radiosurgery for trigeminal neuralgia. In: Winn HR, Youmans JR, editors. Youmans and Winn neurological surgery: fully, searchable text online. Philadelphia, PA: Elsevier; 2017. p. 5486–505.
6. Leksell L. Sterotaxic radiosurgery in trigeminal neuralgia. Acta Chir Scand. 1971;137:311–4.
7. Pollock BE, Phuong LK, Foote RL, Stafford SL, Gorman DA. High-dose trigeminal neuralgia radiosurgery associated with increased risk of trigeminal nerve dysfunction. Neurosurgery. 2001;49:58–62.
8. Brisman R, Mooij R. Gamma knife radiosurgery for trigeminal neuralgia: dose-volume histograms of the brainstem and trigeminal nerve. J Neurosurg. 2000;93(Suppl 3):155–8.
9. Marshall K, Chan MD, McCoy TP, Aubuchon AC, Bourland JD, McMullen KP, et al. Predictive variables for the successful treatment of trigeminal neuralgia with gamma knife radiosurgery. Neurosurgery. 2012;70:566–72.
10. Kondziolka D, Lunsford LD, Flickinger JC, Young RF, Vermeulen S, Duma CM, et al. Stereotactic radiosurgery for trigeminal neuralgia: a multiinstitutional study using the gamma unit. J Neurosurg. 1996;84:940–5.
11. Matsuda S, Serizawa T, Nagano O, Ono J. Comparison of the results of 2 targeting methods in Gamma Knife surgery for trigeminal neuralgia. J Neurosurg. 2008;109(Suppl):185–9.
12. Régis J, Bartolomei F, Metellus P, Rey M, Genton P, Dravet C, et al. Radiosurgery for trigeminal neuralgia and epilepsy. Neurosurg Clin N Am. 1999;10:359–77.
13. Massager N, Lorenzoni J, Devriendt D, Desmedt F, Brotchi J, Levivier M. Gamma knife surgery for idiopathic trigeminal neuralgia performed using a far-anterior cisternal target and a high dose of radiation. J Neurosurg. 2004;100:597–605.
14. Park SH, Hwang SK, Kang DH, Park J, Hwang JH, Sung JK. The retrogasserian zone versus dorsal root entry zone: comparison of two targeting techniques of gamma knife radiosurgery for trigeminal neuralgia. Acta Neurochir. 2010;152:1165–70.

15. Pollock BE, Schoeberl KA. Prospective comparison of posterior fossa exploration and stereotactic radiosurgery dorsal root entry zone target as primary surgery for patients with idiopathic trigeminal neuralgia. Neurosurgery. 2010;67:633–8; discussion 638–639
16. Wang DD, Raygor KP, Cage TA, Ward MM, Westcott S, Barbaro NM, et al. Prospective comparison of long-term pain relief rates after first-time microvascular decompression and stereotactic radiosurgery for trigeminal neuralgia. J Neurosurg. 2017;128:1–10.
17. Régis J, Tuleasca C, Resseguier N, Carron R, Donnet A, Gaudart J, et al. Long-term safety and efficacy of Gamma Knife surgery in classical trigeminal neuralgia: a 497-patient historical cohort study. J Neurosurg. 2016;124:1079–87.
18. Lucas JT, Nida AM, Isom S, Marshall K, Bourland JD, Laxton AW, et al. Predictive nomogram for the durability of pain relief from gamma knife radiation surgery in the treatment of trigeminal neuralgia. Int J Radiat Oncol Biol Phys. 2014;89:120–6.
19. Kondziolka D, Zorro O, Lobato-Polo J, Kano H, Flannery TJ, Flickinger JC, et al. Gamma Knife stereotactic radiosurgery for idiopathic trigeminal neuralgia. J Neurosurg. 2010;112:758–65.
20. Petit JH, Herman JM, Nagda S, DiBiase SJ, Chin LS. Radiosurgical treatment of trigeminal neuralgia: evaluating quality of life and treatment outcomes. Int J Radiat Oncol Biol Phys. 2003;56:1147–53.
21. Maesawa S, Salame C, Flickinger JC, Pirris S, Kondziolka D, Lunsford LD. Clinical outcomes after stereotactic radiosurgery for idiopathic trigeminal neuralgia. J Neurosurg. 2001;94:14–20.
22. Young RF, Vermeulen SS, Grimm P, Blasko J, Posewitz A. Gamma Knife radiosurgery for treatment of trigeminal neuralgia: idiopathic and tumor related. Neurology. 1997;48:608–14.
23. Pollock BE, Phuong LK, Gorman DA, Foote RL, Stafford SL. Stereotactic radiosurgery for idiopathic trigeminal neuralgia. J Neurosurg. 2002;97:347–53.
24. Mousavi SH, Niranjan A, Huang MJ, Laghari FJ, Shin SS, Mindlin JL, et al. Early radiosurgery provides superior pain relief for trigeminal neuralgia patients. Neurology. 2015;85:2159–65.
25. Brisman R, Khandji AG, Mooij RBM. Trigeminal nerve-blood vessel relationship as revealed by high-resolution magnetic resonance imaging and its effect on pain relief after gamma knife radiosurgery for trigeminal neuralgia. Neurosurgery. 2002;50:1261–6; discussion 1266–1267
26. Régis J, Metellus P, Hayashi M, Roussel P, Donnet A, Bille-Turc F. Prospective controlled trial of gamma knife surgery for essential trigeminal neuralgia. J Neurosurg. 2006;104:913–24.
27. Berger I, Nayak N, Schuster J, Lee J, Stein S, Malhotra NR. Microvascular decompression versus stereotactic radiosurgery for trigeminal neuralgia: a decision analysis. Cureus. 2017;9:e1000.
28. Zorro O, Lobato-Polo J, Kano H, Flickinger JC, Lunsford LD, Kondziolka D. Gamma knife radiosurgery for multiple sclerosis-related trigeminal neuralgia. Neurology. 2009;73:1149–54.
29. Tuleasca C, Carron R, Resseguier N, Donnet A, Roussel P, Gaudart J, et al. Multiple sclerosis-related trigeminal neuralgia: a prospective series of 43 patients treated with gamma knife surgery with more than one year of follow-up. Stereotact Funct Neurosurg. 2014;92:203–10.
30. Matsuda S, Nagano O, Serizawa T, Higuchi Y, Ono J. Trigeminal nerve dysfunction after Gamma Knife surgery for trigeminal neuralgia: a detailed analysis. J Neurosurg. 2010;113(Suppl):184–90.
31. Flickinger JC, Pollock BE, Kondziolka D, Phuong LK, Foote RL, Stafford SL, et al. Does increased nerve length within the treatment volume improve trigeminal neuralgia radiosurgery? A prospective double-blind, randomized study. Int J Radiat Oncol Biol Phys. 2001;51:449–54.

Part IV

Other Treatment Options for Trigeminal Neuralgia

Cryotherapy for Trigeminal Neuralgia

Ashish Bindra

Key Points

- Cryotherapy causes reversible ablation of nerves thereby providing pain relief
- It is yet another modality for treatment of trigeminal neuralgia; may be used as an adjuvant therapy to medical management
- It is a simple and repeatable procedure with less reported side-effects

Introduction

Cryotherapy means treating with cold. Cold causes reversible ablation of peripheral nerves and provide pain relief. The utility of cooling therapy is known since the time of Hippocrates [1]. James Arnott (1797–1883), an English physician, first published work on use of cold for treatment of pain in breast, skin and uterine cancers. Due to makeshift agents used and vague technique of delivery, the modality remained less popular. Irving S Cooper, a neurosurgeon contributed enormously to cryosurgery by designing a cryoprobe utilizing liquid nitrogen. The probe could attain a temperature of −196 °C and was used to freeze thalamus for treatment of Parkinson's disease and other movement disorders [2]. Thereafter, liquid nitrogen became popular and was used across many specialities. The advent of cryoprobe enabled clinicians to precisely control area of lesion and also minimise destruction to neighbouring tissues. Lloyd et al. (1976) used it to treat facial pain and found its utility in patients

A. Bindra (✉)
Department of Neuroanaesthesiology and Critical Care, All India Institute of Medical Sciences (AIIMS), New Delhi, India

G. P. Rath (ed.), *Handbook of Trigeminal Neuralgia*,
https://doi.org/10.1007/978-981-13-2333-1_23

with TGN [3]. Thereafter, its benefit for relieving chronic facial pain especially due TGN was reported by many clinicians [4, 5].

Mechanism of Action

Cryotherapy in neuralgia works by freezing nerve cells and thus, blocking transmission of pain. The mechanism of action of Cryotherapy can be divided into three parts:

1. **Heat transfer/heat exchange**: The heat between target area and cryogenic agent is exchanged due to temperature gradient between the two. The common agents used to produce sub-zero temperatures are liquid nitrogen, nitrous oxide, and carbon dioxide. Liquid nitrogen has a boiling point of −196 °C, nitrous oxide −88 °C, carbon dioxide −79 °C [6]. The agent can be delivered by spraying, direct application with a cotton applicator, or with a cryoprobe. When liquid nitrogen is sprayed on the target tissue, it gets evaporated immediately and heat exchange occurs due to evaporation. With a cryoprobe, the heat transfer occurs through conduction.
2. **Cell Injury**: Due to reduction of temperature, the cellular water gets converted to ice crystals resulting in cell injury. Cellular hyperosmolarity prevents cellular freezing unless temperature reaches −5 to −10 °C. Freezing causes concentration of extracellular solutes and results in creation of osmotic gradient which further adds to cellular injury.
3. **Inflammation** is the result of cellular destruction. With use of cryotherapy there occurs minimal tissue destruction and thus, limited inflammation and neuroma formation. Cryogenic nerve injury is characterized by axonal and myelin sheath disintegration causing type-2 nerve injury (Wallerian degeneration). Since the epineurium, perineurium, and endoneurium are preserved, nerve regeneration occurs. Histological changes are suggestive of axonal degeneration within 7 days of treatment. Axonal regeneration occurs at a rate of 1–1.5 mm/week and takes weeks to months for proximal neurons to regenerate. Progressive axonal regeneration and recovery to normal structures is seen around 24 weeks post treatment [6]. With completion of re-innervation symptoms may recur.

Technique

Cryogenic agents such as liquid nitrogen, liquid nitrous oxide, or carbon dioxide decrease temperature of the target tissue when delivered by means of spraying, direct application, or through a cryoprobe. **Cryoprobe** is a hand-held device used to deliver compressed liquid gas via small gauge needle (cryo-needle) for reversible nerve lesioning. The cryoprobe using liquid nitrogen can attain a temperature of −190 °C at its tip. The cryoprobe is based on Thompson Joule principle and depending upon the agent used could attain a temperature up to −50 °C to −70 °C. It is a double lumen probe with an outer and an inner cannula. The outer cannula is connected to a gas source and cryogen is delivered down it at a high pressure (600–800 psi). Since gas under pressure escapes through a small lumen near the probe tip, there is massive fall in pressure to about 10–15 psi which leads to cooling and formation of an ice ball at the tip of probe. The size of ice ball varies from 3.5 to 6 mm depending upon the size of needle used and type of tissue being cryolyzed. In general, bigger the probe, bigger is the ice ball, and more is the area of damage. The inner cannula is used to vent out the gas. Usually14 G/18 G probes are used for cryoneurolysis [6].

The cryoprobe designed for neurolysis has an inbuilt nerve stimulator and thermistor for nerve localization and monitoring target temperature at its tip. After cryolesioning probe should be withdrawn only after thawing to avoid nerve avulsion. The use of introducer needle is recommended to avoid damage to cryo-needle. Both hand held and console tethered cryprobes are available in the market. The hand piece of the probe should remain vertical while lesioning. The freeze and thaw cycles depend upon the type of probe and agent used. Manufacturer's recommendations should be followed. The system is cooled down for about 40 s and the subsequent freezing is done lasting for 90 s. After a period of thawing the freezing is to be repeated.

Application in Trigeminal Neuralgia

Patients with TGN, in whom high dose of drugs has caused considerable side effects can benefit from cryotherapy [7–9]. It produces a reliable, prolonged and reversible trigeminal nerve block without aggravation of symptoms. It is a simple and repeatable procedure in patients who want to avoid major surgery or when the latter is contra-indicated. Cryotherapy has been shown to produce symptomatic pain relief due to primary as well as secondary TGN [10].

Open dissection, percutaneous and transmucosal approach has been used for Cryo-lesioning of trigeminal nerve and its peripheral branches. Cryo-lesioning has been done for inferior alveolar, buccal, mental, lingual, auriculotemporal, supraorbital, and infraorbital nerves. Peripheral branches of trigeminal nerve at the infraorbital or mandibular foramen can be frozen without exposing the nerve or damaging the surrounding tissue. The cryoprobe can be applied in the same way as a needle for a nerve block at infraorbital or mental foramen, by an intraoral approach. Computed tomography (CT) guided imaging has been used to precisely position the probe near the central nerve endings. Dar et al. documented use of CT guidance and treatment of secondary TGN using percutaneous cryoablation. Palliative cryoablation procedures were performed under CT guidance in recurrent head and neck malignancy [10].

The procedure is not painful and does not require general anesthesia. Reduction of pain is seen within 5 days and complete pain relief is seen in another 15 days. The dose of drugs can be titrated down after the procedure. The duration of pain relief in patients receiving cryosurgery may range from 0 days to 4 years [11]. In various case reports average duration of pain relief is limited to 6–12 months. Small duration of procedure, small wound, lesser rate of infection and ease of technique makes it user friendly. Recurrence and partial benefit is common but due to lack of side effects the procedure can be repeated as many times as required [12]. The reported adverse effects include temporary sensory loss, migration of pain to another division of trigeminal nerve and oedema. Cryotherapy comes with inherent risk of trauma during needle placement, bleeding, infection and nerve damage. Since cryotherapy produces type 2 nerve injury, it is less likely to result in neuroma formation, hyperalgesia, deafferentation pain. However, allodynia, hypersensitivity after cryolysis has been reported by few. Anesthesia is seen in few cases though the sensations return back within 6 months.

Other treatment modalities for TGN have their own risk benefit profile. Microvascular decompression (MVD) is an invasive procedure requiring craniotomy and subsequent risk of severe adverse effects. These are relatively contraindicated in elderly patients and in patients with multiple comorbidities. Cryosurgery can be a complement to the medical management in such patients. Electrocoagulation is known to produce side effects like permanent loss of sensation, motor disturbances, including weakness of the masseter muscle and palsy of muscles innervated by oculomotor nerve. Glycerol injection and gamma knife radiosurgery have minimal such problems. However, glycerol injection may be associated with development of deafferentation pain, neuroparalytic keratitis, or anesthesia dolorosa [13]. Though cryotherapy is not associated with significant side effects but its effectiveness has not been proven in large studies. It has been documented only on basis of clinical reports. There are only a few RCTs comparing effectiveness of cryotherapy with other available modalities of treatment.

Conclusion

Although not popular, cryotherapy is one of the promising treatment modalities for TGN. It produces a reliable, prolonged and reversible nerve block without aggravation of symptoms. It is a simple and repeatable procedure in patients who want to avoid a major neurosurgery or where the surgery is contra-indicated. However, the effectiveness of cryosurgical procedures need to be evaluated with large RCTs.

References

1. Cooper SM, Dawber RP. The history of cryosurgery. J R Soc Med. 2001;94:196–201.
2. Cooper IS. Cryogenic surgery. A new method of destruction or extirpation of benign or malignant tissues. N Engl J Med. 1963;263:741–9.
3. Lloyd JW, Barnard JDW, Glynn CJ. Cryoanalgesia. A new approach to pain relief. Lancet. 1976;2:932–4.
4. Nally FF. A 22-year study of paroxysmal trigeminal neuralgia in 211 patients with a 3-year appraisal of the role of cryotherapy. Oral Surg. 1984;58:17–23.
5. Zakrzewska JM, Nally FF, Flint SR. Cryotherapy in the management of paroxysmal trigeminal neuralgia. J Maxillofac Surg. 1986;14:4–7.
6. Ilfeld BM, Preciado J, Trescot AM. Novel cryoneurolysis device for the treatment of sensory and motor peripheral nerves. Expert Rev Med Devices. 2016;13:713–25.

7. Zakrzewska JM. Cryotherapy in the management of paroxysmal trigeminal neuralgia. J Neurol Neurosurg Psychiatry. 1987;50:485–7.
8. Pradel W, Hlawitschka M, Eckelt U, Herzog R, Koch K. Cryosurgical treatment of genuine trigeminal neuralgia. Br J Oral Maxillofac Surg. 2002;40:244–7.
9. De Coster D, Bossuyt M, Fossion E. The value of cryotherapy in the management of trigeminal neuralgia. Acta Stomatol Belg. 1993;90:87–93.
10. Dar SA, Love Z, Prologo JD, Hsu DP. CT-guided cryoablation for palliation of secondary trigeminal neuralgia from head and neck malignancy. J NeuroIntervent Surg. 2013;5:258–63.
11. Lindström M, Thuring N. The value of cryosurgery in the management of trigeminal neuralgia: a systematic review. In: Malmo University Electronic Publishing. http://hdl.handle.net/2043/14392
12. Poon CY. Cryotherapy in the management of trigeminal neuralgia: a review of the literature and report of three cases. Singap Dent J. 2000;23:49–55.
13. Parmar M, Sharma N, Modgill V, Naidu P. Comparative evaluation of surgical procedures for trigeminal neuralgia. J Maxillofac Oral Surg. 2013;12:400–9.

Neuromodulation in Trigeminal Neuralgia

Ritesh Lamsal and Girija Prasad Rath

Key Points

- Standard treatment of trigeminal neuralgia (TGN) is based on pharmacological and surgical methods, and both modalities have variable success rates
- Neuromodulation has added a new spectrum in the management of TGN and involves the use of several upcoming technologies and diverse range of devices
- Underlying mechanisms of neuromodulation are incompletely understood, but rapidly evolving

Introduction

The treatment of classical trigeminal neuralgia (TGN) has traditionally revolved around the use of antiepileptic drugs (AEDs), and surgery in drug-refractory cases. Both techniques have variable degrees of success and recurrence is a common theme in many patients. Further, pharmacotherapy and surgery are not devoid of adverse effects or complications. There are also some studies that show good results with other techniques, like ablative procedures [1] and botulinum injections [2], but there are wide differences in their applications, dosing protocols, long-term efficacy, and overall acceptance across various institutes. Neuromodulation is an exciting prospect that utilizes advanced technologies using electrical or chemical methods, targeting either neural stimulation or inhibition, in order to restore normal

R. Lamsal · G. P. Rath (✉)
Department of Neuroanaesthesiology and Critical Care Neurosciences Centre, All India Institute of Medical Sciences, New Delhi, India

G. P. Rath (ed.), *Handbook of Trigeminal Neuralgia*,
https://doi.org/10.1007/978-981-13-2333-1_24

Table 1 Broad classification of neuromodulation techniques

• Central Techniques
– Transcranial Magnetic Stimulation – Motor Cortex Stimulation – Deep Brain Stimulation – Spinal Cord (cervico-medullary) Stimulation
• Peripheral Techniques
– Transcutaneous Electric Nerve Stimulation – Trigeminal Nerve Stimulation – Gasserian Ganglion Stimulation

neurological function. Neuromodulation techniques to treat TGN are still in nascent stages, with considerable room to evolve and improve. However, there are promising results from some preliminary studies. A broad classification scheme of various neuromodulation techniques is presented in Table 1.

Transcranial Magnetic Stimulation

Transcranial magnetic stimulation (TMS) is a method employing magnetic fields to stimulate neural tissue. First described by Barker and colleagues in 1985, TMS uses implantable electrodes or electromagnetic coils to deliver painless electromagnetic pulses to modulate cortical function [3]. The earliest descriptions of TMS use were in movement disorders [4] and migraine [5], but it has recently been studied in several pain syndromes, including TGN, and other painful trigeminal neuropathies. Lefaucheur and colleagues [6] first demonstrated transient pain relief in drug-refractory TGN with repetitive magnetic stimulation of the precentral motor cortex. There are also some reports of long-lasting pain relief with multiple sessions of TMS [7, 8]. Larger trials are needed to ascertain whether TMS can be effective in providing clinically significant pain-relief in patients with TGN.

Motor Cortex Stimulation

The earliest descriptions of motor cortex stimulation (MCS) for treating central neuropathic pain were published by Tsubokawa and colleagues in the 1990s [9, 10]. MCS is a more invasive modality than TMS using electrodes placed either in the epidural or subdural space, to directly stimulate the motor cortex. MCS works in a multifactorial manner to attenuate mechanical allodynia, such as by inducing neuronal changes in the anterior cingulate gyrus, regulation of synaptic plasticity, and by altering the levels of various neural proteins [11]. Meyerson reported a 60–90% pain reduction in a series of five patients of TGN using MCS [12]. In another case series, all patients with MCS electrodes reported of satisfactory initial pain control, and nearly 60% patients experienced long-term pain relief (mean follow-up: 33 months) [13]. There is also one report of MCS use in a 3-year old child with secondary TGN, with nearly 75% reduction in pain after the procedure [14]. A small, randomized, cross-over trial of MCS in patients with refractory peripheral neuropathic pain, which included TGN, reported a significant reduction in mean visual analogue scale (VAS) scores at one year [15]. It must be noted that all these evidences are either from case reports, case series or small-sized trials. There are also reports of complications like seizures (12%), infections (5%), hardware-related problems (5%) and epidural/subdural hematoma after MCS-electrode implantation, all of which merit careful consideration. The European Academy of Neurology (EAN) guidelines in 2016, made a 'weak recommendation' for the use of MCS in TGN because of the paucity of high-quality supportive evidence [16].

Deep Brain Stimulation

Deep Brain Stimulation (DBS) technology uses a battery-powered, neurostimulating, implantable pulse generator (IPG), which stimulates electrodes placed in targeted cerebral structures, using extension cables that connect IPG to the electrodes. Since its inception nearly 30 years ago [17], DBS has been extensively studied in neurology, most notably in the treatment of movement disorders (essential tremor, Parkinson's disease) and epilepsy. Depending on the site and proposed mechanism of pain, the location of electrode implantation have varied from the thalamus, periaqueductal gray matter, posterior hypothalamus, internal capsule to the motor cortex [18]. DBS placement is invasive and several adverse effects such as infection, lead displacement, intracranial bleeding, seizure, syncope and even death have been reported [19]. There are only a few case reports and open-label studies evaluating the role of DBS in treating neuropathic pain, largely because of the nature of potential complications, cost-implications and invasiveness of the procedure. The results of studies are mixed; some of the studies have reported limited success, whereas, others have refuted its utility. In a case series of 20 patients with intractable pain that underwent DBS of the posterior hypothalamus, 10 of 16 patients with cluster headache had complete pain relief at 18 months, whereas, none of the three patients with atypical facial pain had any pain relief [20]. In another case series, none of the four patients suffering from classical TGN benefited from the procedure (zero response rate), but all five (100%) patients with TGN secondary to multiple sclerosis had good response with DBS placement in the posterior hypothalamus [21]. In light of available evidence, better controlled studies are required to provide reliable information on DBS efficacy in treating TGN.

Spinal Cord Stimulation

Spinal cord stimulation (SCS) uses a device to deliver electrical stimuli to the spinal cord to modulate chronic pain. The mechanism of pain reduction is believed to be due to alteration of neurochemistry in the dorsal horn, which in turn, suppresses central hyper-excitability [22]. SCS has been used for several decades in the management of complex regional pain syndrome (CRPS), back pain, and leg pain. It has also been explored in the management of craniofacial pain by stimulation of the cervico-medullary junction (CMJ). A retrospective case series reported that seven out of ten patients with post-traumatic trigeminal neuropathy, four of five patients with chronic trigeminal neuropathic pain, and two out of two patients with post-herpetic TGN responded favourably with CMJ stimulation. Another retrospective study reported that mean pain severity reduced by 59% (from 8 to 3.3) in four patients of TGN treated with SCS at CMJ, with satisfactory pain control for a mean of five years (range: 0–4 years) [23]. Even though SCS is an invasive modality with certain inherent risks, there are promising reports of satisfactory pain control in refractory TGN using CMJ stimulation. However, in the absence of any randomized study, it is too early to draw any meaningful conclusion.

Transcutaneous Electric Nerve Stimulation

Transcutaneous electric nerve stimulation (TENS) is a promising option for the management of TGN. The technique is non-invasive, not expensive, has very few reported side effects, and works by delivering electric current across the intact surface of the skin. TENS is based on the gate-control theory of pain, which states that repetitive activation of large nerve fibres with stimuli like pressure, touch and vibration, facilitate presynaptic inhibition of substantia gelatinosa cells resulting in decreased pain transmission. A study in 30 patients with TGN reported that after 20-min daily application of TENS, for 20–40 days, using a portable TENS machine, the mean VAS score in patients at 3 months significantly decreased from 8.9 to 1.3 [24]. Another prospective study in 31 patients with drug-refractory TGN reported significant improvement in pain in over 80% of the patients using TENS for 3 weeks [25]. Again, similar to several other neuromodulation techniques, there are no large randomized studies assessing the efficacy of TENS to draw substantive conclusions. A Cochrane systematic review in 2017 concluded that the quality of available evidence is too low to effectively state whether TENS is effective in treating neuropathic pain [26].

Peripheral Nerve Stimulation

Peripheral nerve stimulation (PNS) is a modality of pain management based on the same principles of gate-control theory that TENS is based on. In contrast to the non-invasive nature of TENS, PNS makes use of electrodes that are implanted via a minimally invasive surgery and attached to the affected nerve. The use of PNS for several neuropathic pain syndromes such as occipital neuralgia, CRPS, post-traumatic neuralgia, and post-herpetic neuralgia have been well-documented [27]. Several case reports have shown serially-repeated PNS to be effective in decreasing TGN pain [28–31]. In a retrospective series of ten patients with intractable facial pain, eight patients reported of significant and lasting pain relief after permanent PNS placement [32]. Remarkably, the mean VAS scores in these patients decreased from 9.3 to 0.75 (range 0–3) [32]. Similar findings were found in a cohort study, where seven out of eight patients with refractory TGN responded to PNS; mean pain intensity on VAS decreased by over 70%. However, in the largest reported retrospective study on PNS till date, more than half the patients (18 of 35) had a poor response to initial trial stimulation and were not considered for permanent PNS electrode placement [33]. In the subset of patients who went on to receive permanent PNS placement, over two-thirds of them had significant pain relief [33]. The overall results from these studies are mixed and findings are not conclusive. Large prospective studies are required to firmly establish PNS in the management of TGN. Until then, its use in TGN continues to be off-label.

Other Modalities

Apart from the modalities discussed above, there are also reports of the use of other neuro-modulating techniques such as transcranial direct current stimulation [34], percutaneous trigeminal ganglion intervention [35], peripheral cryotherapy [36], laser irradiation [37], and streptomycin-lidocaine injections [38]. Most of the literature for these modalities are available in the form of case reports and small series of cases. The available evidences are weak, large studies are absent, and no concrete conclusions can be made.

Conclusion

The use of neuromodulation techniques to alleviate TGN pain is an exciting field, even though it is still in its early stages. Strong recommendations cannot be made, given the paucity of supportive evidence. However, with advancement in our understanding of the pathophysiology of craniofacial pain, coupled with technological evolution, the future of neuromodulation holds a lot of promise to extenuate the agonies of TGN.

References

1. Udupi BP, Chouhan RS, Dash HH, Bithal PK, Prabhakar H. Comparative evaluation of percutaneous retrogasserian glycerol rhizolysis and radiofrequency thermocoagulation techniques in the management of trigeminal neuralgia. Neurosurgery. 2012;70:407–12; discussion 12–3
2. Bohluli B, Motamedi MH, Bagheri SC, Bayat M, Lassemi E, Navi F, et al. Use of botulinum toxin A for drug-refractory trigeminal neuralgia: preliminary report. Oral Surg Oral Med Oral Pathol Oral Radiol Endod. 2011;111:47–50.
3. Barker AT, Jalinous R, Freeston IL. Non-invasive magnetic stimulation of human motor cortex. Lancet. 1985;1:1106–7.
4. Cantello R. Applications of transcranial magnetic stimulation in movement disorders. J Clin Neurophysiol. 2002;19:272–93.

5. Lipton RB, Dodick DW, Silberstein SD, Saper JR, Aurora SK, Pearlman SH, et al. Single-pulse transcranial magnetic stimulation for acute treatment of migraine with aura: a randomised, double-blind, parallel-group, sham-controlled trial. Lancet Neurol. 2010;9:373–80.
6. Lefaucheur JP, Drouot X, Nguyen JP. Interventional neurophysiology for pain control: duration of pain relief following repetitive transcranial magnetic stimulation of the motor cortex. Neurophysiol Clin. 2001;31:247–52.
7. Khedr EM, Kotb H, Kamel NF, Ahmed MA, Sadek R, Rothwell JC. Longlasting antalgic effects of daily sessions of repetitive transcranial magnetic stimulation in central and peripheral neuropathic pain. J Neurol Neurosurg Psychiatry. 2005;76:833–8.
8. Zaghi S, DaSilva AF, Acar M, Lopes M, Fregni F. One-year rTMS treatment for refractory trigeminal neuralgia. J Pain Symptom Manage. 2009;38:e1–5.
9. Tsubokawa T, Katayama Y, Yamamoto T, Hirayama T, Koyama S. Chronic motor cortex stimulation for the treatment of central pain. Acta Neurochir Suppl (Wien). 1991;52:137–9.
10. Tsubokawa T, Katayama Y, Yamamoto T, Hirayama T, Koyama S. Chronic motor cortex stimulation in patients with thalamic pain. J Neurosurg. 1993;78:393–401.
11. Cha M, Um SW, Kwon M, Nam TS, Lee BH. Repetitive motor cortex stimulation reinforces the pain modulation circuits of peripheral neuropathic pain. Sci Rep. 2017;7:7986.
12. Meyerson BA, Lindblom U, Linderoth B, Lind G, Herregodts P. Motor cortex stimulation as treatment of trigeminal neuropathic pain. Acta Neurochir Suppl (Wien). 1993;58:150–3.
13. Raslan AM, Nasseri M, Bahgat D, Abdu E, Burchiel KJ. Motor cortex stimulation for trigeminal neuropathic or deafferentation pain: an institutional case series experience. Stereotact Funct Neurosurg. 2011;89:83–8.
14. Delavallee M, Rooijakkers H, Koerts G, Raftopoulos C. Motor cortex stimulation in a three-year-old child with trigeminal neuropathic pain caused by a malignant glioma in the cerebellopontine angle: case report. Neurosurgery. 2011;69:E494–6.
15. Lefaucheur JP, Drouot X, Cunin P, Bruckert R, Lepetit H, Creange A, et al. Motor cortex stimulation for the treatment of refractory peripheral neuropathic pain. Brain. 2009;132:1463–71.
16. Cruccu G, Garcia-Larrea L, Hansson P, Keindl M, Lefaucheur JP, Paulus W, et al. EAN guidelines on central neurostimulation therapy in chronic pain conditions. Eur J Neurol. 2016;23:1489–99.
17. Benabid AL, Pollak P, Louveau A, Henry S, de Rougemont J. Combined (thalamotomy and stimulation) stereotactic surgery of the VIM thalamic nucleus for bilateral Parkinson disease. Appl Neurophysiol. 1987;50:344–6.
18. Perlmutter JS, Mink JW. Deep brain stimulation. Annu Rev Neurosci. 2006;29:229–57.
19. Leone M. Deep brain stimulation in headache. Lancet Neurol. 2006;5:873–7.
20. Broggi G, Franzini A, Leone M, Bussone G. Update on neurosurgical treatment of chronic trigeminal autonomic cephalalgias and atypical facial pain with deep brain stimulation of posterior hypothalamus: results and comments. Neurol Sci. 2007;28(Suppl 2):S138–45.
21. Franzini A, Messina G, Cordella R, Marras C, Broggi G. Deep brain stimulation of the posteromedial hypothalamus: indications, long-term results, and neurophysiological considerations. Neurosurg Focus. 2010;29:E13.
22. Oakley JC, Prager JP. Spinal cord stimulation: mechanisms of action. Spine (Phila PA 1976). 2002;27:2574–83.
23. Chivukula S, Tempel ZJ, Weiner GM, Gande AV, Chen CJ, Ding D, et al. Cervical and cervicomedullary spinal cord stimulation for chronic pain: efficacy and outcomes. Clin Neurol Neurosurg. 2014;127:33–41.
24. Singla S, Prabhakar V, Singla RK. Role of transcutaneous electric nerve stimulation in the management of trigeminal neuralgia. J Neurosci Rural Pract. 2011;2:150–2.
25. Yameen F, Shahbaz NN, Hasan Y, Fauz R, Abdullah M. Efficacy of transcutaneous electrical nerve stimulation and its different modes in patients with trigeminal neuralgia. J Pak Med Assoc. 2011;61:437–9.
26. Gibson W, Wand BM, O'Connell NE. Transcutaneous electrical nerve stimulation (TENS) for neuropathic pain in adults. Cochrane Database Syst Rev. 2017;9:Cd011976.

27. Stidd DA, Wuollet AL, Bowden K, Price T, Patwardhan A, Barker S, et al. Peripheral nerve stimulation for trigeminal neuropathic pain. Pain Physician. 2012;15:27–33.
28. Abd-Elsayed AA, Grandhi R, Sachdeva H. Effective management of trigeminal neuralgia by neurostimulation. Ochsner J. 2015;15:193–5.
29. Weiner RL, Garcia CM, Vanquathem N. A novel miniature, wireless neurostimulator in the management of chronic craniofacial pain: preliminary results from a prospective pilot study. Scand J Pain. 2017;17:350–4.
30. Simpson BA, Nannapaneni R. Trigemino-cervical neuropathic pain relieved by serially repeated peripheral nerve field stimulation without tolerance: case report. Neuromodulation. 2017;20:383–5.
31. Slavin KV, Colpan ME, Munawar N, Wess C, Nersesyan H. Trigeminal and occipital peripheral nerve stimulation for craniofacial pain: a single-institution experience and review of the literature. Neurosurg Focus. 2006;21:E5.
32. Klein J, Sandi-Gahun S, Schackert G, Juratli TA. Peripheral nerve field stimulation for trigeminal neuralgia, trigeminal neuropathic pain, and persistent idiopathic facial pain. Cephalalgia. 2016;36:445–53.
33. Ellis JA, Mejia Munne JC, Winfree CJ. Trigeminal branch stimulation for the treatment of intractable craniofacial pain. J Neurosurg. 2015;123:283–8.
34. Fricova J, Englerova K, Rokyta R. Noninvasive transcranial direct current stimulation (tDCS) for the treatment of orofacial pain. Neuro Endocrinol Lett. 2016;37:368–72.
35. Van Buyten JP. Trigeminal ganglion stimulation. Prog Neurol Surg. 2015;29:76–82.
36. Poon CY. Cryotherapy in the management of trigeminal neuralgia: a review of the literature and report of three cases. Singapore Dent J. 2000;23:49–55.
37. Falaki F, Nejat AH, Dalirsani Z. The effect of low-level laser therapy on trigeminal neuralgia: a review of literature. J Dent Res Dent Clin Dent Prospects. 2014;8:1–5.
38. Kreiner M. Use of streptomycin-lidocaine injections in the treatment of the cluster-tic syndrome. Clinical perspectives and a case report. J Craniomaxillofac Surg. 1996;24:289–92.

Botulinum Toxin for Trigeminal Neuralgia

Arunmozhimaran Elavarasi and Vinay Goyal

Key Points

- Trigeminal neuralgia (TGN) is a chronic painful condition, which compromises the quality of life of the patient
- Botulinum neurotoxin (BoNT) is an alternative to surgery in patients with drug-refractory TGN
- BoNT relieves symptoms and reduces drug requirement in patients with drug-refractory TGN
- BoNT can be useful in reducing drug-related adverse effects

Introduction

The American Academy of Neurology and the European Federation of Neurological Societies (AAN/EFNS) guidelines for the management of trigeminal neuralgia (TGN) suggest anticonvulsant medications as first line therapy; the surgical options utilized drug-refractory cases [1]. However, many patients are refractory to drugs, and surgical treatment may not be feasible owing to associated comorbid illnesses. Interventional procedures on the peripheral trigeminal nerve or on the Gasserian ganglion may not always be possible because of the unavailability of skilled

A. Elavarasi
Department of Neurology, Jawaharlal Institute of Postgraduate Medical Education and Research (JIPMER), Puducherry, India

V. Goyal (✉)
Department of Neurology, Neurosciences Centre, All India Institute of Medical Sciences (AIIMS), New Delhi, India

G. P. Rath (ed.), *Handbook of Trigeminal Neuralgia*,
https://doi.org/10.1007/978-981-13-2333-1_25

practitioners. Botulinum neurotoxin (BoNT) is a promising mode of treatment, which can help such patients and provide pain relief.

Botulinum Toxin and Preparations

BoNT is produced by the anerobic bacteria Clostridium botulinum. The toxin has seven antigenic serotypes (A to G) and causes motor paralysis and botulism [2]. Out of the seven BoNTs, botulinum neurotoxin type-A is widely used for therapeutic purposes. Commonly available products include—onabotulinum toxin-A (Botox), incobotulinum toxin-A (Xeomin) and abobotulinum toxin-A (Dysport). Rimabotulinum toxin-B (Myobloc) is less commonly used. Botox and Xeomin are nearly equipotent with a conversion ratio of 1:1, and can be used interchangeably [3]. However, for Dysport, a ratio of 3:1 is used for conversion to Botox (3 units of Dysport = 1 unit of Botox) [4].

Mechanism of Action of BoNT

Botulinum toxin acts at the neuromuscular junction by inhibiting acetylcholine (Ach) release, thereby decreasing muscle fiber activity [5]. Specifically, BoNTs bind to various sites on the 'soluble *N*-ethylmaleimide-sensitive factor Attachment protein Receptor' (SNARE) proteins, which are essential for fusion of Ach vesicles to the plasma membrane and subsequent exocytosis of Ach into the neuromuscular junction [6]. However, nociceptive properties of the toxin are due to its effects on peripheral and central pain pathways. BoNT has been postulated to act through inhibition of various neurotransmitters, such as calcitonin gene related peptide (CGRP), substance P, glutamate, as well as the expression of transient receptor potential vanilloid 1 [7].

Role of BoNT in Pain Management

When first introduced, BoNT was primarily used to relieve symptoms in conditions with increased muscle tone or activity such as dystonia, strabismus and spasticity. In these conditions, the toxin inhibits the release of Ach, thereby decreasing neuromuscular transmission, and reducing muscle tone. Early studies found that in patients with painful cervical dystonia who were given BoNT injections, there was improvement of pain symptoms much earlier than dystonia-related features [8]. This led to a surge of studies investigating its effects in myriad painful conditions like myofascial pain, neuropathic pain syndromes, as well as other painful musculoskeletal conditions. In 2002, Michelo et al. [9] first reported significant relief of pain with BoNT in a patient with TGN. Subsequently, various reports have highlighted the efficacy of BoNT in alleviating pain attributed to TGN [10–12].

Safety and Efficacy

Clinical data on BoNT use is available in patients of different age groups. It is safe and equally effective across all ages. Even though some early animal studies have indicated reduction in fetal weight and decreased fetal ossification with BoNT use in pregnancy, there is only one published literature till date, that has reported spontaneous abortion in a pregnant patient who received BoNT [13]. Whether the abortion was clearly attributed to BoNT is not known. On the other hand, there are several case-reports of pregnant patients who have been treated with botulinum toxin without any adverse effects in the new-born [14, 15]. However, the drug continues to be labelled as risk-category C in pregnancy [13], and it is best to avoid using it in pregnant patients, unless newer recommendations for its use are amended. In any case of accidental injection in a pregnant lady, careful follow-up of the fetus is warranted. Similarly, BoNT is contraindicated in patients who have neuromuscular diseases.

Routes of Administration

BoNT is usually given as subcutaneous or submucosal injections at trigger points or areas representing most significant pain. The injection may be given as a fixed dose or calculated as per the area involved. In general, subcutaneous injection in the facial region is the commonest technique. However, there is always a risk of inadvertent intramuscular injections because facial muscles are very superficial. This may lead to temporary weakness or paralysis of facial muscles. There are some studies where the drug was deliberately given intramuscularly in the masseter or temporalis muscles, and have demonstrated better results compared submucosal injection [16, 17]. It is hypothesized that when injected intramuscularly, the toxin effectively travels in a retrograde direction through the axons of the motor branch of the trigeminal nerve due to its rich blood supply, leading to better efficacy compared to submucosal injections [17]. In one study, BoNT was directly injected into the maxillary and mandibular branches of the trigeminal nerve at the pterygopalatine fossa [12]. There is no common consensus for BoNT injections, with different routes, doses and duration-protocols followed by pain physicians, based on their personal experiences or institutional practices.

BoNT Use in TGN

There are four published randomized controlled trials (RCTs) examining the effect of BoNT in the treatment of TGN (Table 1) [16, 18–20]. A meta-analysis of these four RCTs, published in 2016 [21] found that the patients receiving BoNT had better response to treatment as well as lower frequency of paroxysms per day, as compared to placebo [21]. Various small, open-labelled trials studied use of BoNT in TGN. In a small study, injection of BoNT into maxillary and mandibular nerve roots was found be effective in providing 50% pain relief in 90% patients, and complete pain relief in 44% patients, at 6 months [12].

Table 1 Randomized trials in the treatment of TGN with BoNT

Study	Participants	Intervention	Outcome
Shehata et al. [19] Randomized single blinded placebo controlled	20 patients with TGN diagnosed according to IHS ICHD 2 criteria and less than 50% reduction in VAS or paroxysm frequency during the last 3 months with appropriate drugs	BoNT 5U (0.1 mL) or 0.9% saline (0.1 mL) in each trigger point, injection also into masseter muscle in mandibular branch involvement	Reduction in VAS at 12 weeks was by 6.5 in BoNT group and 0.3 for placebo. Significant decrease in the number of acute medications and an increase in quality of life
Wu et al. [18] Randomized, double blind, placebo controlled	42 patients with TGN diagnosed according to ICHD 2 criteria and failure of last treatment at baseline (pain intensity mean score 4; mean attack frequency 4 per day)	75U of BoNT-A (1.5 mL) or 1.5 mL of 0.9% saline	VAS scores and mean attack frequency at 12 weeks was significantly lower in the BoNT group compared to placebo. 68% patients in BoNT group responded with more than 50% reduction in VAS compared to only 15% patients in placebo
Zuniga et al. [16] Randomized double blind placebo controlled	36 patients with TGNs defined by Classification of Chronic Pain: Descriptions of Chronic Pain Syndromes and Definitions of Pain Terms	50U of BoNT in 1 mL of 0.9% saline or 1 mL of 0.9% saline 10U in masseter muscle in V3 involvement	Three months after the injection, average VAS score of those treated with BoNT was 4.75 vs. 6.94 in those treated with placebo; *t* test $P = 0.01$)
Zhang et al. [20] Randomized double blind placebo controlled study	84 patients with TGN diagnosed according to ICHD II and >18 years), with failure of recent treatment (pain intensity mean score ≥4; mean attack frequency ≥4 per day; course >4 months)	1 mL of saline containing 50U of BoNT vs. 1 mL of plain saline injected in 20 points (0.05 mL/point)	3 months after the injection, statistically significant differences were observed in the average VAS score for subjects treated with BoNT compared to placebo

TGN Trigeminal neuralgia, *BoNT* Botulinum neurotoxin, *IHS* International Headache Society, *ICHD* International Classification of Headche Disorders, *VAS* Visual analog score

Author Experience and Institutional Protocol

The authors have an extensive experience of using BoNT in TGN. It has been believed that there is a significant reduction in the need for medications such as carbamazepine or gabapentin after BoNT treatment. Antiepileptic medications have a variety of unwanted effects and de-escalation of therapy helps in mitigating several of these adverse effects. In our Institute, patients are assessed for baseline pain intensity measured on the 11-point visual analogue scale (VAS, 0–10). BoNT-A is diluted (100 IU BOTOX, Allergan, USA in 2.5 mL normal saline), and intradermal or submucosal (if pain is over oral mucosa) injections are given using a tuberculin syringe with 30G needle. The injection sites are selected based on the patients' narrative of most painful areas and specific trigger zones. Total painful area is calculated after demarcating it on the face. BoNT is injected in doses of 3 IU/cm^2 of pain surface area. None of our patient had suffered severe facial weakness using this protocol. Hence, it is believed to be a simple, safe and effective protocol which can be easily adopted elsewhere.

Conclusion

There is ample evidence to support of use of BoNT in TGN. This drug can drastically improve the quality of life and increase productivity of the individual by alleviating excruciating pain symptoms of TGN. Even though there is no comparative study of BoNT with neurosurgical decompression or other interventional modalities, it is a safe and effective modality of treatment. With careful explanation on potential side-effects, this treatment modality may be offered to all patients with drug-refractory symptoms, unless specific contraindications exist.

References

1. Cruccu G, Gronseth G, Alksne J, Argoff C, Brainin M, Burchiel K, Nurmikko T, Zakrzewska JM, American Academy of Neurology Society, European Federation of Neurological Society. AAN-EFNS guidelines on trigeminal neuralgia management. Eur J Neurol. 2008;15:1013–28.
2. Macdonald TE, Helma CH, Shou Y, Valdez YE, Ticknor LO, Foley BT, et al. Analysis of Clostridium botulinum serotype E strains by using multilocus sequence typing, amplified fragment length polymorphism, variable-number tandem-repeat analysis, and botulinum neurotoxin gene sequencing. Appl Environ Microbiol. 2011;77:8625–34.
3. Scaglione F. Conversion ratio between Botox(R), Dysport(R), and Xeomin(R) in clinical practice. Toxins (Basel). 2016;8:pii:E65.
4. Walker TJ, Dayan SH. Comparison and overview of currently available neurotoxins. J Clin Aesthet Dermatol. 2014;7:31–9.
5. Simpson LL. The origin, structure, and pharmacological activity of botulinum toxin. Pharmacol Rev. 1981;33:155–88.
6. Verderio C, Grumelli C, Raiteri L, Coco S, Paluzzi S, Caccin P, et al. Traffic of botulinum toxins A and E in excitatory and inhibitory neurons. Traffic. 2007;8:142–53.
7. Oh HM, Chung ME. Botulinum toxin for neuropathic pain: a review of the literature. Toxins (Basel). 2015;7:3127–54.
8. Colhado OC, Boeing M, Ortega LB. Botulinum toxin in pain treatment. Rev Bras Anestesiol. 2009;59:366–81.
9. Micheli F, Scorticati MC, Raina G. Beneficial effects of botulinum toxin type a for patients with painful tic convulsif. Clin Neuropharmacol. 2002;25:260–2.
10. Allam N, Brasil-Neto JP, Brown G, Tomaz C. Injections of botulinum toxin type a produce pain alleviation in intractable trigeminal neuralgia. Clin J Pain. 2005;21:182–4.
11. Zuniga C, Diaz S, Piedimonte F, Micheli F. Beneficial effects of botulinum toxin type A in trigeminal neuralgia. Arq Neuropsiquiatr. 2008;66:500–3.
12. Turk Boru U, Duman A, Boluk C, Coskun Duman S, Tasdemir M. Botulinum toxin in the treatment of trigeminal neuralgia: 6-month follow-up. Medicine (Baltimore). 2017;96:e8133.
13. Morgan JC, Iyer SS, Moser ET, Singer C, Sethi KD. Botulinum toxin A during pregnancy: a survey of treating physicians. J Neurol Neurosurg Psychiatry. 2006;77:117–9.
14. Paul M. Controversy: botulinum toxin in pregnancy. J Cutan Aesthet Surg. 2009;2:4–5.

15. Newman WJ, Davis TL, Padaliya BB, Covington CD, Gill CE, Abramovitch AI, et al. Botulinum toxin type A therapy during pregnancy. Mov Disord. 2004;19:1384–5.
16. Zuniga C, Piedimonte F, Diaz S, Micheli F. Acute treatment of trigeminal neuralgia with onabotulinum toxin A. Clin Neuropharmacol. 2013;36:146–50.
17. Wu C, Xie N, Liu H, et al. A new target for the treatment of trigeminal neuralgia with botulinum toxin type A. Neurol Sci. 2018;39:599–602.
18. Wu CJ, Lian YJ, Zheng YK, Zhang HF, Chen Y, Xie NC, et al. Botulinum toxin type A for the treatment of trigeminal neuralgia: results from a randomized, double-blind, placebo-controlled trial. Cephalalgia. 2012;32:443–50.
19. Shehata HS, El-Tamawy MS, Shalaby NM, Ramzy G. Botulinum toxin-type A: could it be an effective treatment option in intractable trigeminal neuralgia? J Headache Pain. 2013;14:92.
20. Zhang H, Lian Y, Ma Y, Chen Y, He C, Xie N, et al. Two doses of botulinum toxin type A for the treatment of trigeminal neuralgia: observation of therapeutic effect from a randomized, double-blind, placebo-controlled trial. J Headache Pain. 2014;15:65.
21. Morra ME, Elgebaly A, Elmaraezy A, Khalil AM, Altibi AM, Vu TL, et al. Therapeutic efficacy and safety of botulinum toxin A therapy in trigeminal neuralgia: a systematic review and meta-analysis of randomized controlled trials. J Headache Pain. 2016;17:63.

Neural Prolotherapy for Trigeminal Neuralgia

Ankur Khandelwal and Girija Prasad Rath

Key Points

- Neural prolotherapy or perineural injection therapy (PIT) involves subcutaneous injections of low concentration of 5% dextrose or 5% mannitol to heal injured superficial nerves
- The anti-nociceptive property of PIT is attributed to dextrose induced antagonism of pro-inflammatory Transient Receptor Potential Cation Channel V1 (TRPV1) receptors expressed on nerve membrane
- It has the advantages of minimal invasiveness, cost effectiveness, and low side-effect profile
- It has the potential to be utilized in trigeminal neuralgia as a stand-alone or adjunctive treatment to either reduce or eliminate the need for medications and surgery

Introduction

Trigeminal neuralgia (TGN) is a syndrome of unilateral, lancinating, paroxysmal, stabbing orofacial neuropathic pain, confined to the distribution of one or more of the branches of the trigeminal nerve. Most of the patients respond well to pharmacotherapy; carbamazepine and oxcarbazepine being the first line treatment. Surgical options are available if medications are no longer effective or tolerated. Microvascular decompression, gamma knife radiosurgery, and percutaneous rhizotomies are most promising surgical alternatives [1, 2]. Recently, neural

A. Khandelwal · G. P. Rath (✉)
Department of Neuroanaesthesiology and Critical Care Neurosciences Centre,
All India Institute of Medical Sciences, New Delhi, India

G. P. Rath (ed.), *Handbook of Trigeminal Neuralgia*,
https://doi.org/10.1007/978-981-13-2333-1_26

prolotherapy has been described in relation to the management of TGN. It is also known as **perineural injection therapy (PIT)** and is one of the latest advancements in regenerative medicine. First described by Dr. Paul Pybus and Dr. Roger Wyburn-Mason, PIT targets neurogenic inflammation in subcutaneous nerves that potentially generates pain [3, 4]. It was further refined by Dr. John Lyftgoft using hypertonic dextrose injection, which provided substantial pain control in a series of 300 Achilles tendinopathy [5]. He described the technique as subcutaneous injections of 0.5–1 mL of hypertonic dextrose and local anesthetic at each tender point alongside the affected tendon and thereafter repeating the treatment at weekly intervals. This was a departure from the traditionally described prolotherapy in which a more concentrated proliferant is injected directly into the enthesis of an affected structure causing discomfort and increased pain at the time of injection and in the immediate following few days.

In recent years, a variety of neurogenic pain syndromes, other than TGN, such as complex regional pain syndrome, carpal tunnel syndrome, diabetic neuropathy, Morton's neuroma, post herpetic neuralgia, post-surgical pain, reflex sympathetic dystrophy and fibromyalgia have been treated with neural prolotherapy. Prolotherapy is also used to treat pain due to musculoskeletal injuries including shoulder, knee, elbow, neck and low back, ankle, temporal mandibular joint (TMJ), and many other conditions [6–16].

Procedure

Typically, prolotherapy involves shallow injections of low concentration of 5% dextrose or 5% mannitol under the skin to heal injured superficial nerves. The procedure is typically performed with a 27 G ½ inch needle. Approximately 1–2 mL of solution is injected into each site. The number of injections varies with the area and symptoms to be treated. As this alternate approach merely involves injection into the subcutaneous tissue and with a lesser gauge needle, there is significantly less discomfort to the patient [5, 12]. It has been termed a "regenerative" injection therapy due to the properties of healing damaged intra-articular and peri-articular soft tissues, including cartilage, ligaments, tendons, and fascial structures and promoting nerve repair [17].

Concept of Neuralgia and Neural Prolotherapy

Tissue injury or injury to nerves by stretching, constricting, or cutting them (such as after surgery or due to tight muscle spasms), activate a receptor on nerves called Transient Receptor Potential Cation Channel V1 (TRPV1), also known as the capsaicin, vanilloid or chili pepper receptor. Upregulation of TRPV-1 receptors results in release of pro-inflammatory chemicals such as Calcitonin Gene-Related Peptide (CGRP) and substance P that causes inflammation, swelling, burning painful sensations (neuropathic pain) and chronic nerve dysfunction [18, 19]. Meng and colleagues demonstrated that TRPV1 stimulation mediated the release of CGRP which in turn increased the excitability of trigeminal sensory neurons in brainstem slices via CGRP1 receptors [20]. In a study by Urano and colleagues, rats were subjected to partial infraorbital nerve ligation to mimic the nerve damage seen in TGN. The goal was to induce heat and mechanical sensitivity and evaluate the effectiveness of a TRPV1 antagonist in reducing this sensitivity. This study found that heat hyperalgesia was decreased with TRPV1 antagonism and that TRPV1 expression in large neurons in the trigeminal ganglia was increased [21]. It is postulated that dextrose and mannitol inhibit TRPV1 nerve receptors, preventing this inflammatory cascade and restoring normal nerve function. Dextrose blocks nociceptive pain. Sensation to touch remains intact unlike lignocaine which blocks both mechanosensitive and insensitive nociceptors leading to numbness [7].

Review of Literature

Conaway et al reported of a 63 year old female complaining of 13 years of burning pain on the face and scalp due to V1 branch TGN after neurosurgical intervention for cerebral aneurysm. Counter analgesics and tramadol-acetaminophen provided little relief. Initial treatment with osteopathic manipulation provided symptomatic relief for a few hours. Hence, neural prolotherapy was performed with two injections one week apart, and the third injection 12 weeks later. The technique involved identification of the supraorbital foramen by palpation and then the pattern of her pain was followed in a linear fashion superiorly across the forehead and scalp based on knowledge of anatomy and the patients' area of reported pain. 3 mL syringes with a 0.5 inch needle were prepared with a solution of 5% dextrose in water (D5W). The tender points were each injected with 0.5 mL of solution, at a 45° angle, 0.5–1 cm deep, and approximately 1–2 cm apart. The solution was injected while withdrawing the needle so as to create a skin bleb. On each subsequent treatment the area of the pain was progressively reduced and subsequently, injection of fewer sites was required. After three treatments with neural prolotherapy, the patient experienced complete resolution of pain due to TGN [6].

In another report, a 70-year-old male presented with a 15-year history of pain due to TGN involving all three divisions on right side, and the pain was refractory to pharmacologic treatment. The patient was then placed in the left lateral decubitus position and the right side of the face was treated utilizing a neural prolotherapy technique. Approximately 15 injections were provided to the distribution of the 3 involved branches of the trigeminal nerve. A 27 G ½ inch needle was used to inject a 5% dextrose solution into the subcutaneous tissues. Approximately 1–2 mL was injected in each area. After one treatment of neural prolotherapy the patient reported 5 months of complete resolution of symptoms. A second treatment provided the patient another 10 months of pain relief [7].

Complications

- Infection and tissue injury: With proper technique the risk is minimal to none
- Local swelling and bruising
- Mild transient pain

Contraindications

- **Absolute Contraindications:** Joint or skin infection, active flare of a rheumatological condition, allergy to corn, and use of immunosuppressive medications.
- **Relative Contraindications:** Acute fracture, acute gout, bleeding disorders, and use of anticoagulants [22].

Conclusion

Neural prolotherapy has the potential to be utilized in TGN and any other neuralgia of an accessible peripheral nerve. It may serve as a stand-alone or adjunctive treatment to either reduce or eliminate the need for medications and surgery. As the technique is minimally invasive with a low side effect profile, it could be considered prior to surgical intervention and perhaps even before long term pharmacotherapy is initiated. Large randomized controlled trials is the need of the hour for the validation and acceptability of this neural regenerative therapy.

References

1. Al-Quliti KW. Update on neuropathic pain treatment for trigeminal neuralgia. The pharmacological and surgical options. Neurosciences (Riyadh). 2015;20:107–14.
2. Feller L, Khammissa RAG, Fourie J, Bouckaert M, Lemmer J. Postherpetic neuralgia and trigeminal neuralgia. Pain Res Treat. 2017;2017:1681765.
3. Reeves KD, Lyftogt J. Prolotherapy: regenerative injection therapy. In: Waldman SD, editor. Pain management. 2nd ed. Philadelphia, PA: Saunders (Elsevier); 2011. p. 1027–44.
4. Geppetti P, Holzer P. Neurogenic inflammation. Boca Raton, FL: CRC Press; 1996.
5. Lyftogt J. Subcutaneous prolotherapy for achilles tendinopathy: the best solution? Aust Musculoskeletal Med. 2007;122:107–9.
6. Conaway E, Browning B. Neural prolotherapy for neuralgia. J Prolotherapy. 2014;6:928–31.
7. Itkin A. Treatment of trigeminal neuralgia utilizing neural prolotherapy: a case report. J Prolotherapy. 2016;8:961–5.
8. Thor JA, Mohamed Hanapi NH, Halil H, Suhaimi A. Perineural injection therapy in the management of complex regional pain syndrome: a sweet solution to pain. Pain Med. 2017;18:2041–5.
9. Wu YT, Ho TY, Chou YC, et al. Six-month efficacy of perineural dextrose for carpal tunnel syndrome: a prospective, randomized, double-blind, controlled trial. Mayo Clin Proc. 2017;92:1179–89.
10. Hauser RA, Steilen DR, Fisher P. Upper cervical instability of traumatic origin treated with dextrose prolotherapy: a case report. J Prolotherapy. 2015;7:932–5.

11. Hauser RA, Feister WA. Treatment of basal thumb osteoarthritis: a retrospective study of dextrose prolotherapy injections as an alternative treatment. J Prolotherapy. 2013;5:913–21.
12. Lyftogt J. Subcutaneous prolotherapy treatment of refractory knee, shoulder and lateral elbow pain. Aust Musculoskeletal Med. 2007;12:110–2.
13. Weglein AD. Neural prolotherapy. J Prolotherapy. 2011;3:639–43.
14. Wheaton MT, Jensen N. The ligament injury-osteoarthritis connection: the role of prolotherapy in ligament repair and the prevention of osteoarthritis. J Prolotherapy. 2011;3:790–812.
15. Harris GR. Effective treatment of chronic pain by the integration of neural therapy and prolotherapy. J Prolotherapy. 2010;2:377–86.
16. Hauser RA, Gruen KA. The use of prolotherapy in the treatment of chronic overuse shoulder and neck pain, neurogenic pain and hip degeneration in an incomplete C4-C5 spinal cord injury patient. J Prolotherapy. 2009;1:166–71.
17. DM DC, Cortazzo MH. Regenerative medicine in the field of pain medicine: prolotherapy, platelet-rich plasma, and stem cell therapy—theory and evidence. Tech Reg Anesth Pain Manag. 2011;15:74–80.
18. Alawi K, Keeble J. The paradoxical role of the transient receptor potential vanilloid 1 receptor in inflammation. Pharmacol Ther. 2010;125:181–95.
19. Geppetti P, Nassini R, Materazzi S, Benemei S. The concept of neurogenic inflammation. BJU Int. 2008;101(Suppl 3):2–6.
20. Meng J, Ovsepian SV, Wang J, et al. Activation of TRPV1 mediates calcitonin gene-related peptide release, which excites trigeminal sensory neurons and is attenuated by a retargeted botulinum toxin with anti-nociceptive potential. J Neurosci. 2009;29:4981–92.
21. Urano H, Ara T, Fujinami Y, Hiraoka BY. Aberrant TRPV1 expression in heat hyperalgesia associated with trigeminal neuropathic pain. Int J Med Sci. 2012;9:690–7.
22. Rabago D, Nourani B. Prolotherapy for osteoarthritis and tendinopathy: a descriptive review. Curr Rheumatol Rep. 2017;19:34.

Complementary Medicine in Trigeminal Neuralgia

Rajeeb Kumar Mishra and Girija Prasad Rath

> **Key Points**
> - Trigeminal neuralgia (TGN) is a chronic debilitating painful condition
> - Complimentary medicine is an adjunct to standard treatment options like pharmacotherapy and surgical interventions
> - Complementary medicine acts synergistically with conventional treatment in reducing painful episodes of TGN

Introduction

Trigeminal neuralgia (TGN) is a chronic debilitating condition characterized by recurrent attacks of lancinating pain in the distribution of the trigeminal nerve. Carbamazepine is the initial drug of choice for treating TGN [1]; however, several other drugs, including antidepressants may provide pain relief in some cases. Neurosurgical treatment may be helpful in treating drug-refractory cases. Apart from pharmacotherapy and surgical interventions, several complementary therapies provide additional benefit.

Role of Complementary Therapy in Public Health Management

When non-mainstream practice is used together with conventional medicine, it is considered as 'complementary' [2]. Complementary healing practices represent a vast and yet unrealized sector of public health systems [3]. Different

R. K. Mishra · G. P. Rath (✉)
Department of Neuroanaesthesiology and Critical Care Neurosciences Centre, All India Institute of Medical Sciences, New Delhi, India

G. P. Rath (ed.), *Handbook of Trigeminal Neuralgia*,
https://doi.org/10.1007/978-981-13-2333-1_27

complementary therapies such as acupuncture, and transcutaneous electrical nerve stimulation (TENS) have been tried for the management of TGN. PainShield is a novel method of ultrasonology based treatment aimed at reducing the intensity of painful episodes. Nutritional therapy constitutes certain vitamins and minerals, which help in reducing pain severity. Homeopathy, biofeedback, psychotherapy, yoga and meditation are other modalities to control the psychic component of pain and thus, reduce the intensity and frequency of painful episodes. Utility of some of these modalities have been elaborated further in this chapter.

Acupuncture

Acupuncture is a form of alternative medicine and is a key component of ancient Chinese medicine. It involves placement of small and thin needles in specific body locations, thereby helping to alleviate pain. It is the most commonly used alternative therapy for relief of pain, even though there are doubts on its safety and efficacy. Acupuncture is based on the presumption that there are patterns of energy flow (Qi) in the body which are essential for health, and any disruption of this flow leads to disease or pain [4]. It has been believed that acupuncture corrects imbalances of flow at identifiable points close to the skin. The proposed mechanism of analgesic effect of acupuncture is attributed to the augmented plasma levels of mediators such as endorphin, encephalin and serotonin [5]. There are several published reports suggesting acupuncture and electro-acupuncture to be beneficial in TGN. Tian surveyed the literature related to acupuncture treatment for TGN and found encouraging rates of efficacy with regard to pain relief [6]. Yang and colleagues suggested that comprehensive therapy of electro-acupuncture at "qi" acupoints, combined with spinal regulation is a safe and effective method that provides long-term efficacy in TGN compared with oral carbamazepine alone [7]. A pilot study comparing traditional acupuncture to combination of traditional and ear acupuncture for treating headache, TGN, and retro-auricular pain in facial palsy found significant pain relief after the fifth and sixth sessions of acupuncture ($p = 0.021$; $p = 0.025$) [8]. Multiple sessions of I Ching Balance Acupuncture (ICBA) technique has been successfully used to treat medically refractory TGN [9]. Acupuncture practitioners claim that if acupuncture is applied very soon after the onset of the disease condition, it is more effective in curing it.

Transcutaneous Electrical Nerve Stimulation

Transcutaneous electrical nerve stimulation (TENS) produces eletro-analgesia by utilizing the principle of "gate control theory". The analgesic effects of TENS have been attributed to neuromodulation by various proposed mechanisms, such as presynaptic inhibition in the dorsal horn of the spinal cord, endogenous pain control (via endorphins, enkephalins, and dynorphins), direct inhibition of an abnormally excited nerve, and restoration of afferent input. The application of TENS is vast;

it is effective in reducing both acute and chronic pain using low-voltage electric currents through the intact surface of skin. The TENS unit is a small, programmable, battery-powered equipment consisting of electrodes and an electric-signal generator. The generator delivers trains of stimuli of variable amplitudes, pulse widths, and pulse rates. The optimal setting of the electric stimulus is subjective; three options are available: (i) Conventional TENS using high frequency stimulus (50–100 Hz) with low intensity current, just above threshold (10–30 mA) and at a pulse width of 50–80 μs for 30 min, several times during a day, (ii) Acupuncture-like low frequency stimulus (1–10 Hz) with high intensity current up to the tolerable limits of the patients, and (iii) Pulsed/Burst TENS using low-intensity stimuli firing at high frequency recurrent bursts discharge at 1–2 Hz. The use of TENS in TGN looks promising with several advantages like being inexpensive, safe, self-administrable, and without any major side-effects. In a study out of 31 patients of TGN, 26 (83.7%) improved significantly with application of TENS and five (16.3%) patients remained unresponsive to this therapy. The authors suggested that TENS is effective, easy to use, and constant mode of therapy is slightly better than the burst mode [10]. In another study, considerable decrease in pain rating as defined by visual analogue scale (VAS) score and verbal pain scores were observed [11].

Therapeutic Ultrasound (PainShield)

Ultrasound is a form of mechanical energy, which is transmitted to the biological tissues as acoustic pressure waves at very high frequencies. Conventionally, therapeutic ultrasound is in the frequency and intensity ranges of 1–3 MHz and 0.2–1 W/cm^2, respectively. The long duration ultrasound may overheat the adjoining tissue and damage it. However, ultrasound is beneficial when applied at low intensity and low frequency ranges (KHz instead of MHz).

The PainShield is a portable, battery-operated, low intensity, low frequency ultrasound (LILFU) device. It provides low energy of therapeutic ultrasound to create a slow-release effect on the targeted area, thereby allowing prolonged and more effective treatment. The surface acoustic waves (SAWs), unlike traditional ultrasound, provides a wide treatment zone, and hence, enables longer treatment durations, while keeping the total energy exposure of the body at a safe level [12, 13]. When applied over bony surfaces such as the forehead, the SAWs travel the entire skull including the brain tissues. Hence, the root entry zone of the trigeminal nerve and all its branches are exposed to LILFU/SAW.

The PainShield (NanoVibronix Inc, Farmingdale, NY) generates this slow-energy via a reusable/disposable adhesive patch, placed along the distribution of the trigeminal nerve (Fig. 1), with continuous-wave ultrasound at a frequency of 90 kHz, and an acoustic power of 0.07 W/cm^2. The patch incorporates a thin, flexible transducer that delivers ultrasound energy to the underlying biological tissues to relieve pain and induce soft tissue healing [14]. The patients are usually suggested to use during sleep every day and to remove the patch when they wake up. The device is programmed to switch on and off for 30 min each, for a total duration of 8 h.

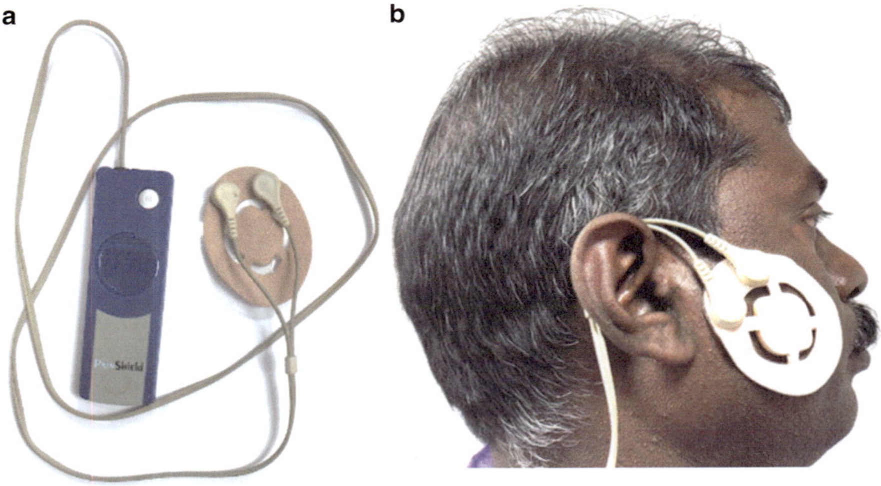

Fig. 1 PainShield with disposable adhesive patch (**a**); patient using the patch/device (**b**)

The actuator is applied over bony prominences, such as the zygomatic arch for maxillary (V2) neuralgia, and on the lower jaw for mandibular (V3) neuralgia.

Therapeutic ultrasound using PainShield seems to be a noble technique for pain relief or reduction of medication in patients with TGN. In view of increased interest on its beneficial effects, PainShield as a technology needs further evaluation.

Vitamins and Nutritional Therapy

Several nutritional elements including vitamins, fish oils and antioxidants may be helpful in relieving TGN pain. Fresh fruits such as apples, oranges, mangoes, and peaches are rich in these essential mineral supplements and help to strengthen the nerves. Antioxidants like ascorbyl palmitate and lemon fish oil, which are sometimes prescribed in rheumatoid arthritis, have been shown to benefit patients with drug-refractory TGN [15]. Vitamin C decreases spontaneous pain in patients with post-herpetic neuralgia [16] and hence, may be of some benefit in TGN. Another interesting article depicts the role of B vitamins in the treatment of induced infraorbital neuropathy in rats [17]. Repeated administrations of B1 (thiamine), B6 (pyridoxine) and B12 vitamins prevented heat hyperalgesia after infraorbital nerve injury, but only B12 and B6 treatments attenuated cold and mechanical hyperalgesia, respectively [17]. These findings suggest B vitamins might constitute complementary adjuncts to conventional therapy in patients suffering from trigeminal neuropathic pain.

Biofeedback Therapy

Biofeedback is a treatment modality in chronic pain disorders that comprises of patients' physiological data analyzed in real time via sensors placed on the body. Biofeedback process enables an individual to learn how to change physiological activity for the purposes of improving health and performance [18]. Biofeedback along with diaphragmatic breathing technique, cognitive behavioral therapy, and stress management help to reduce the level of pain as the patient learns to control emotions and cope with lifestyle difficulties [19].

Homeopathy

Homeopathy is a highly controversial alternative method to control both acute flare ups and the chronic disease condition. One study suggests that homeopathic treatment is an effective and safe method in the treatment of idiopathic TGN. Although it is a small population study, the results are encouraging. The authors found overall reductions of more than 60% in pain intensity using homeopathic treatment during a four-month follow up period [20].

Yoga and Meditation

Exercise and diet play important roles to achieve good health of individuals. Deep breathing exercise may help some patients to decrease pain of TGN. Various yoga and meditation techniques have been suggested to cure neurological disorders. There are no large studies validating the role of yoga or breathing exercises in decreasing TGN pain; however, proponents of these techniques advocate that they be performed regularly to achieve notable improvement in symptoms.

Psychotherapy

Chronic pain syndromes are frequently associated with psychiatric abnormalities. There is an increased attention towards temporal association of TGN with psychiatric problems [21, 22]. Wu and colleagues carried out a population based retrospective cohort study to explore this relationship [23]. They concluded that TGN might increase the risk of newly diagnosed psychiatric problems such as depression, anxiety, and sleep disorders, which affect the quality of life. Emotional stress is another factor which may aggravate the pain perception of TGN. Hence, psychological counselling is necessary as a part of multi-pronged approach to the management of this chronic condition.

Conclusion

TGN is a chronic distressing illness which needs a multimodal approach to achieve satisfactory pain control. Along with the conventional therapies, complementary medicines can have a positive impact on the patient's overall health. Futuristic therapeutic models might include complementary medicines; however, more research is needed in this field to understand and substantiate its role.

References

1. Wiffen PJ, McQuay HJ, Moore RA. Carbamazepine for acute and chronic pain. Cochrane Database Syst Rev. 2005:CD005451.
2. National center for complementary and integrative health. Complementary, alternative, or integrative health: what's in a name? Available at: https://nccih.nih.gov/health/integrative-health#cvsa. Accessed Jan 10, 2018.
3. Silenzio VMB. What is the role of complementary and alternative medicine in public health? Am J Public Health. 2002;92:1562–4.
4. Ernst E, Lee MS, Choi TY. Acupuncture: does it alleviate pain and are there serious risks? A review of reviews. Pain. 2011;152:755–64.
5. Cabýoglu MT, Ergene N, Tan U. The mechanism of acupuncture and clinical applications. Int J Neurosci. 2006;116:115–25.
6. Tian LF. A survey on acupuncture treatment of trigeminal neuralgia. J Tradit Chin Med. 2010;30:68–76.
7. Yang JX, Zhang JP, Yu JC, Han JX. Clinical research of primary trigeminal neuralgia treated with electroacupuncture at qi streets acupoints combined with spinal regulation therapy. Zhongguo Zhen Jiu. 2014;34:763–8.
8. Ahn CB, Lee SJ, Lee JC, Fossion JP, Sant'Ana A. A clinical pilot study comparing traditional acupuncture to combined acupuncture for treating headache, trigeminal neuralgia and retro-auricular pain in facial palsy. J Acupunct Meridian Stud. 2011;4:29–43.
9. Kotlyar A. Treatment of facial pain with I Ching balance acupuncture. Med Acupunct. 2017;29:405–10.
10. Yameen F, Shahbaz NN, Hasan Y, Fauz R, Abdullah M. Efficacy of transcutaneous electrical nerve stimulation and its different modes in patients with trigeminal neuralgia. J Pak Med Assoc. 2011;61:437–9.
11. Singla S, Prabhakar V, Singla RK. Role of transcutaneous electric nerve stimulation in the management of trigeminal neuralgia. J Neurosci Rural Pract. 2011;2:150–2.
12. Uhlemann C, Heinig B, Wollina U. Therapeutic ultrasound in lower extremity wound management. Int J Low Extrem Wounds. 2003;2:152–7.
13. Adahan HM, Sharon H, Siev-Ner I. A sound solution to tendonitis: healing tendon tears with a novel low-intensity, low-frequency surface acoustic ultrasound patch. PMR. 2010;2:685–7.
14. Adahan HM, Yacov I, Siev-Ner I, Alexander B. A sound solution for trigeminal neuralgia. (Conference Paper); 7th Congress of the European Federation of IASP Chapters (EFIC) 2011;Vol 3
15. Carmichael A. PA and fish oil. Br Dent J. 2012;212:356–7.
16. Kapoor S. Vitamin C for attenuating postherpetic neuralgia pain: an emerging treatment alternative. J Headache Pain. 2012;13:591.
17. Kopruszinski CM, Reis RC, Chichorro JG. B vitamins relieve neuropathic pain behaviours induced by infraorbital nerve constriction in rats. Life Sci. 2012;91:1187–95.
18. Institute for chronic pain. What is biofeedback? Available at: https://www.instituteforchronicpain.org/treating-common-pain/what-is-pain management/biofeedback. Accessed Jan 10, 2018.

19. Sime ALCSW. Case study of trigeminal neuralgia using neurofeedback and peripheral biofeedback. J Neurother. 2004;8:59–71.
20. Mojaver YN, Mosavi F, Mazaherinezhad A, Shahrdar A, Manshaee K. Individualized homeopathic treatment of trigeminal neuralgia: an observational study. Homeopathy. 2007;96:82–6.
21. Zakrzewska JM. Multi-dimensionality of chronic pain of the oral cavity and face. J Headache Pain. 2013;14:37.
22. Hals EKB, Stubhaug A. Mental and somatic co-morbidities in chronic orofacial pain conditions: pain patients in need of multiprofessional team approach. Scand J Pain. 2011;2:153–4.
23. Wu TH, Hu LY, Lu T, Chen PM, Chen HJ, Shen CC, et al. Risk of psychiatric disorders following trigeminal neuralgia: a nationwide population-based retrospective cohort study. J Headache Pain. 2015;16:64.

Part V

Special Scenario with Trigeminal Neuralgia

Trigeminal Neuralgia in Multiple Sclerosis

Nitasha Mishra

Key Points
- Trigeminal neuralgia (TGN) occurs in 1–2% of patients suffering from multiple sclerosis (MS)
- The characteristic of pain is similar to classical TGN, except for a high probability of bilateral presentation
- TGN in MS is believed to be due to demyelination of the sensory fibers of trigeminal nerve
- Pharmacotherapy is the first-line of management; baclofen and misoprostol have shown promising results
- Surgical procedures have been found to offer better outcome in terms of pain relief in some patients

Introduction

Multiple sclerosis (MS) is the most prevalent chronic inflammatory disease of the central nervous system (CNS), affecting more than 2 million people worldwide [1]. It is punctuated by fully or partially reversible episodes of neurologic disability, usually lasting for days or weeks. The typical syndrome at presentation include, but is not limited to, monocular visual loss due to optic neuritis, limb weakness or sensory loss due to transverse myelitis, double vision due to brain-stem

N. Mishra (✉)
Department of Anaesthesiology, All India Institute of Medical Sciences (AIIMS), Bhubaneswar, India

G. P. Rath (ed.), *Handbook of Trigeminal Neuralgia*,
https://doi.org/10.1007/978-981-13-2333-1_28

dysfunction, or ataxia due to a cerebellar lesion [2]. The association of TGN and multiple sclerosis (MS) has been well-known since the end of the nineteenth century [3]; a strong association has been suggested with a 20-fold higher prevalence of TGN in this group compared to the general population [4]. A systematic review [5] suggested a prevalence of 3.8% of TGN in patients with MS. Patients of TGN due to MS have been found to have a mean age 5.5 year less than those suffering from idiopathic TGN [6].

Clinical Features

The clinical manifestations of TGN in patients with MS are the same as for other types. There are reports, which suggest that the attacks may have atypical features like 'prolonged background pain' [7–9]. Sandell and colleagues [9] observed that patients initially present with episodic pain. Other authors mention that the background pain was not related to presence or absence of demyelination in the trigeminal nerve [10]. It is also suggested that the pain gradually becomes more atypical as multiple divisions of the nerve are involved, and 6% might eventually present with bilateral facial pain [11]. It is generally believed that MS precedes TGN; however, several case-series report TGN as the first symptom, with intervals of 5–10 years before another symptom of MS is manifested [11–13]. No correlation has been observed between the extent of MS plaques and the severity of clinical manifestations of TGN [14, 15]. There is also lack of data as to whether periods of remission occur in patients of MS with TGN.

Pathophysiology of TGN in MS

TGN in patients of MS is considered to be related to a demyelination phenomenon involving the sensory fibers of trigeminal nerve, either within the nerve root, or less commonly, at the brainstem [16, 17]. In case of MS, a plaque of demyelination encompasses the root entry zone (REZ) of the trigeminal nerve in the pons [18]. Love and Coakham [17] demonstrated that demyelination is found to extend along the proximal part of the trigeminal nerve root and, in some cases, right up to its junction with the peripheral nervous system. Additionally, several studies describe the association of a neurovascular conflict in a minority of patients with MS [12, 19–21].

Management

A variety of pharmacological and surgical treatment options for TGN have been described that are effective and widely used. The general recommendation is to start with medical therapy and consider surgical procedures in patients, who are refractory to pharmacotherapy.

Medical Management

The evidence for pharmacologic management of TGN in MS is based on open label studies with small numbers and a high risk of bias. Due to lack of appropriate data, it is difficult to advise how the pain of TGN in MS should be managed. Hence, the same medical management may be suggested, as used for patients with non-MS TGN. Antiepileptic drugs (AEDs) are the first line of pharmacotherapy for all types of pain in MS. These include carbamazepine or oxcarbazepine as first-line agents, and lamotrigine, baclofen, gabapentin, and pregabalin as second-line drugs [22, 23]. Jawahar et al. [24] opined that AEDs are effective for non-TGN pain in MS patients; even though there are reports of some tolerable side effects. Carbamazepine use can lead to side effects, both on hepatic and hematopoietic functions. In some patients, it can impair cerebellar and general motor function leading to weakness, ataxia, dizziness, and nystagmus, which can be very troublesome in patients with MS [25].

Lamotrigine is a new generation AED; its action is mediated by blockade of sodium channels. It produces similar effects like carbamazepine and phenytoin in membrane hyperpolarization. In one study, a total of 28 patients with MS-TGN were treated with lamotrigine, with complete relief of pain observed in 20 patients and partial relief in one patient [26, 27]. Use of lamotrigine may lead to milder side-effects on the CNS than carbamazepine or phenytoin. It has been observed that when MS patients were switched from treatment with carbamazepine to lamotrigine, some of them experienced significant improvement of neurological conditions [27].

Two drugs used more frequently in patients with MS-TGN than in other patients with TGN, are **baclofen** and **misoprostol**. Baclofen is a γ-amino-butyric acid-β receptor agonist and mainly used for spasticity. Its site of action is mostly at the presynaptic level [28]. With centrally acting muscle relaxant action, this drug is particularly helpful in MS patients, although side-effects like hypoesthenia and muscle weakness may occur. Reder and Arnason reported successful use of misoprostol in patients with MS-related TGN [8]. The rationale was misoprostol can inhibit T-lymphocyte functions and consequently, decrease their inflammatory activity in MS plaques by increasing intracellular levels of cyclic adenosine monophosphate (cAMP). In another study, 14 of the 18 patients with refractory TGN showed a reduction in frequency and intensity of pain with the use of misoprostol [29]. Pfau et al. [30] reported successful use of misoprostol in three cases of treatment-resistant TGN in patients with MS, with fewer side effects compared to other drugs.

Surgical Management

Various surgical procedures are offered for the treatment of TGN in MS patients, however, none of them have been proven superior in terms of acute pain relief. There are only small case series reporting treatment outcomes in patients with MS, with a general tendency toward lesser efficacy in this population. Most authors recommend the use of Gasserian ganglion blockade unless a definitive vascular compression of the trigeminal nerve is identified on imaging.

Montano and colleagues [31] suggested the overall acute pain relief (APR) rate of MS patients with drug-resistant TGN subjected to different surgical procedures was 91.8 ± 5.8%, ranging from 85% in patients undergoing gamma-knife radiosurgery (GKRS) to 96% who underwent radiofrequency thermocoagulation (RFT). No procedure offered clearly better results in terms of APR rate. Zakrezewska and colleagues [32] observed that 83.6% of patients had pain relief after various sensory rhizotomy procedures; however, 51.1% experienced recurrence during follow-up. The highest recurrence rate was observed after percutaneous balloon compression (PBC) with pain relief of 60.2 ± 14.4% [31]. This result was significant when compared to GKRS ($p = 0.01$) and microvascular decompression (MVD) ($p = 0.02$). Montano et al. [31] suggested that RFT and MVD offered best chances for being pain-free at follow-up compared to other methods, with least complications following MVD.

Recommendations

The AAN-EFNS guidelines [33] do not prefer one drug over another for management of pain due to TGN in MS patients. It is recommended that before surgical intervention, pharmacological avenues should be thoroughly explored. There is insufficient evidence to support or refute the effectiveness of gabapentin, lamotrigine, misoprostol, and topiramate in treating pain in symptomatic TGN.

- In patients of MS with TGN refractory to medical therapy, early surgical therapy may be considered (Level C).
- Percutaneous procedures on the Gasserian ganglion, gamma knife, and MVD may be considered (Level C).
- MVD may be considered over other surgical techniques to provide the longest duration of pain relief (Level C).

Conclusion

Treatment of MS-related TGN remains a challenge both for neurologists and pain physicians owing to lack of full comprehension of the complex pathogenesis of their association. In absence of high-quality evidence, it is challenging to provide a definitive management plan in such patients. Both pharmacologic and surgical treatment strategies offer pain relief; however, the benefits of treatment are usually short-lived compared to non-MS patients with TGN.

Acknowledgement The author acknowledges contribution of Dr. Sucharita Ray, MD, DM Assistant Professor, Department of Neurology, PGIMER, Chandigarh, India for her valuable inputs in finalizing this manuscript.

References

1. GBD 2015 Neurological Disorders Collaborator Group. Global, regional, and national burden of neurological disorders during 1990–2015: a systematic analysis for the Global Burden of Disease Study 2015. Lancet Neurol. 2017;16:877–97.
2. Brownlee WJ, Hardy TA, Fazekas F, Miller DH. Diagnosis of multiple sclerosis: progress and challenges. Lancet. 2017;389:1336–46.
3. Moulin DE, Foley KM, Ebers GC. Pain syndromes in multiple sclerosis. Neurology. 1988;38:1830–4.
4. Katusic S, Williams DB, Beard CM, Bergstralh E, Kurland LT. Incidence and clinical features of glossopharyngeal neuralgia, Rochester, Minnesota, 1945–1984. Neuroepidemiology. 1991;10:266–75.
5. Foley PL, Vesterinen HM, Laird BJ, Sena ES, Colvin LA, Chandran S, et al. Prevalence and natural history of pain in adults with multiple sclerosis: systematic review and meta-analysis. Pain. 2013;154:632–42.
6. Rushton JG, Olafson RA. Trigeminal neuralgia associated with multiple sclerosis. A case report. Arch Neurol. 1965;13:383–6.
7. Jensen TS, Rasmussen P, Reske-Nielsen E. Association of trigeminal neuralgia with multiple sclerosis: clinical and pathological features. Acta Neurol Scand. 1982;65:182–9.
8. Reder AT, Arnason BG. Trigeminal neuralgia in multiple sclerosis relieved by a prostaglandin E analogue. Neurology. 1995;45:1097–100.
9. Sandell T, Eide PK. The effect of microvascular decompression in patients with multiple sclerosis and trigeminal neuralgia. Neurosurgery. 2010;67:749–53.
10. Abhinav K, Love S, Kalantzis G, Coakham HB, Patel NK. Clinicopathological review of patients with and without multiple sclerosis treated by partial sensory rhizotomy for medically refractory trigeminal neuralgia: a 12-year retrospective study. Clin Neurol Neurosurg. 2012;114:361–5.
11. Mohammad-Mohammadi A, Recinos PF, Lee JH, Elson P, Barnett GH. Surgical outcomes of trigeminal neuralgia in patients with multiple sclerosis. Neurosurgery. 2013;73:941–50.
12. Broggi G, Ferroli P, Franzini A, Nazzi V, Farina L, La Mantia L, et al. Operative findings and outcomes of microvascular decompression for trigeminal neuralgia in 35 patients affected by multiple sclerosis. Neurosurgery. 2004;55:830–8.
13. Linderoth B, Hakanson S. Paroxysmal facial pain in disseminated sclerosis treated by retrogasserian glycerol injection. Acta Neurol Scand. 1989;80:341–6.
14. Kanpolat Y, Berk C, Savas A, Bekar A. Percutaneous controlled radiofrequency rhizotomy in the management of patients with trigeminal neuralgia due to multiple sclerosis. Acta Neurochir. 2000;142:685–9.
15. Hooge JP, Redekop WK. Trigeminal neuralgia in multiple sclerosis. Neurology. 1995;45:1294–6.
16. Love S, Gradidge T, Coakham HB. Trigeminal neuralgia due to multiple sclerosis: ultrastructural findings in trigeminal rhizotomy specimens. Neuropathol Appl Neurobiol. 2001;27:238–44.
17. Love S, Coakham HB. Trigeminal neuralgia: pathology and pathogenesis. Brain. 2001;124:2347–60.
18. Hilton DA, Love S, Gradidge T, Coakham HB. Pathological findings associated with trigeminal neuralgia caused by vascular compression. Neurosurgery. 1994;35:299–303.
19. Broggi G, Ferroli P, Franzini A, Servello D, Dones I. Microvascular decompression for trigeminal neuralgia: comments on a series of 250 cases, including 10 patients with multiple sclerosis. J Neurol Neurosurg Psychiatry. 2000;68:59–64.
20. Meaney JF, Watt JW, Eldridge PR, Whitehouse GH, Wells JC, Miles JB. Association between trigeminal neuralgia and multiple sclerosis: role of magnetic resonance imaging. J Neurol Neurosurg Psychiatry. 1995;59:253–9.
21. Meaney JM, Miles JB. Microvascular decompression for trigeminal neuralgia. J Neurosurg. 1995;83:183–4.

22. Zakrzewska JM, Linskey ME. Trigeminal neuralgia. BMJ Clin Evid. 2014;pii:1207.
23. Zakrzewska JM, Linskey ME. Trigeminal neuralgia. 2015;350:h1238.
24. Jawahar R, Oh U, Yang S, Lapane KL. A systematic review of pharmacological pain management in multiple sclerosis. Drugs. 2013;73:1711–22.
25. Hunter SF, Lim N, Nashville TN. Carbamazepine (CBZ)-induced exacerbation of weakness in severe demyelinating disease. Neurology. 1999;52:135.
26. Lunardi G, Leandri M, Albano C, Cultrera S, Fracassi M, Rubino V, Favale E. Clinical effectiveness of lamotrigine and plasma levels in essential and symptomatic trigeminal neuralgia. Neurology. 1997;48:1714–7.
27. Leandri M, Lundardi G, Inglese M, Messmer-Uccelli M, Mancardi GL, Gottlieb A, Solaro C. Lamotrigine in trigeminal neuralgia secondary to multiple sclerosis. J Neurol. 2000;247:556–8.
28. Kangrga I, Jiang MC, Randic M. Actions of (-)-baclofen on rat dorsal horn neurons. Brain Res. 1991;562:265–75.
29. DMKG study group. Misoprostol in the treatment of trigeminal neuralgia associated with multiple sclerosis. J Neurol. 2003;250:542–5.
30. Pfau G, Brinkers M, Treuheit T, Kretzschmar M, Senturk M, Hachenberg T. Misoprostol as a therapeutic option for trigeminal neuralgia in patients with multiple sclerosis. Pain Med. 2012;13:1377–8.
31. Montano N, Papacci F, CioniRinaDi B, MarioMeglio B. What is the best treatment of drug-resistant trigeminal neuralgia in patients affected by multiple sclerosis? A literature analysis of surgical procedures. Clin Neurol Neurosurg. 2013;115:567–72.
32. Zakrzewska JM, Wu J, Brathwaite TS. A systematic review of the management of trigeminal neuralgia in patients with multiple sclerosis. World Neurosurg. 2011;111:291–306.
33. Cruccu G, Gronseth G, Alksne J, Argoff C, Brainin M, Burchiel K, Nurmikko T, Zakrzewska JM, American Academy of Neurology Society, European Federation of Neurological Society. AAN-EFNS guidelines on trigeminal neuralgia management. Eur J Neurol. 2008;15:1013–28.

Management of Trigeminal Neuralgia During Pregnancy

Bhanu Pratap Swain

Key Points
- Therapeutic armamentarium is grossly depleted when a pregnant woman is afflicted by trigeminal neuralgia (TGN)
- Teratogenicity of commonly used medications and lack of evidence regarding safety of interventional therapies are the common hindrances in the management of TGN during pregnancy
- Carbamazepine, the first-line drug, has teratogenic potential, and should be avoided during pregnancy
- Second-line medications such as lamotrigine and levetiracetam are considered as safer alternatives
- Percutaneous Gasserian ganglion rhizotomy appears to be safe with appropriate precaution for radiation exposure

Introduction

Trigeminal neuralgia (TGN) is a debilitating painful condition which may manifest in pregnant females. It is a medical challenge for pain physicians in view of the limited therapeutic options during pregnancy and lack of adequate knowledge of this unique situation. Utility of the commonly used anti-epileptic drugs (AEDs) is questionable due the risk of teratogenic effect on fetus. Furthermore, there are not enough evidences regarding the safety of interventional procedures employed for

B. P. Swain (✉)
Department of Anesthesiology and Critical Care, Tata Main Hospital, Jamshedpur, Jharkhand, India

G. P. Rath (ed.), *Handbook of Trigeminal Neuralgia*,
https://doi.org/10.1007/978-981-13-2333-1_29

TGN during pregnancy. When such a scenario is encountered, the management needs to be modified considering its implications on both mother and fetus.

Pregnancy and TGN

Barring one case report, our current knowledge of TGN in pregnancy is limited [1]. This makes it difficult for clinicians to outline any management plan. Nonetheless, the diagnosis is essentially clinical and therapeutic options need to be carefully selected considering the current pregnancy. In this context, there are three possible scenarios which might be encountered (as below).

1. A pregnant woman develops TGN for the first time during pregnancy
2. A known patient of TGN controlled with medication plans to conceive
3. A woman conceives unexpectedly who is already on medications for TGN

In the first two scenarios, the women has to be made aware of the possible teratogenic effect of the medications on the fetus and limited data regarding safety of the therapeutic interventions. She should be counselled adequately about the risk and beneficial effects of all possible treatment modalities before instituting or omitting any therapy. The third scenario entails a higher risk to the fetus as the woman continues to take medications until she becomes aware of her pregnancy. By that time, the fetus is already exposed to the harmful effect of the teratogenic drugs during the vulnerable first few weeks of life. Therefore, in this case, once the pregnancy is diagnosed, the offending drug has to be withdrawn immediately, and an alternate treatment strategy has to be initiated. More importantly, the fetus has to be monitored throughout the pregnancy to look for any adverse effect of the drug.

Management Strategy

Pharmacotherapy

Medical management of TGN consists of primarily anticonvulsant drugs (AEDs). Majority of these drugs were initially categorized by US Food and Drug Administration (FDA) under category C or D, which makes it theoretically unsuitable to be used during pregnancy (Table 1). However, since 2015, FDA has replaced the former pregnancy risk letter categories (category A, B, C, D, X) with a new information system to make it more meaningful to the patients and healthcare providers [2]. The Australian system (Therapeutic Goods Administration) has also proposed pregnancy categorization of the drugs (category A, B1, B2, B3, C, D, and X), which is based on the known adverse effects of the drug on the developing fetus, including the potential to cause birth defects, unwanted pharmacological effect at the time of birth and problems later in life [3]. These categorization systems give us a general information about the risk status of the drug which may vary based on the

Table 1 Pregnancy risk category of drugs used in trigeminal neuralgia

Medications	US FDA	AUS TGA
First line therapy		
Carbamazepine	D	D
Oxcarbamazepine	C	D
Second line therapy		
Lamotrigine	C	D
Baclofen	C	B3
Alternative therapy		
Gabapentin	C	B1
Pregabaline	C	B3
Levitiracetam	C	B3
Topiramate	D	D
Botulinum toxin A	C	B3
Other drugs		
Phenytoin	D	D
Clonazepam	–	B3
Amitriptyline	C	C

US FDA: United states Food and Drug Administration
AUS TGA: Therapeutic Goods Administration, Australia

present or future researches. Moreover, the effect of most of the drugs on fetus have been tested in women with epilepsy, where the risk of discontinuing the medication are greater than continuing it. In contrast, TGN or any other chronic pain syndrome does not involve major risk to the life of mother or fetus and hence, the management approach has to be as safe as possible. Nevertheless, it is important to assess various drugs available for treatment of TGN and their safety profile in pregnancy.

Carbamazepine (CBZ) is the first line medication to treat TGN. Although not a potent one, recent studies suggest it be teratogenic [4]. Hence, use of CBZ in pregnancy to manage pain of TGN is discouraged. If at all used, it should be as monotherapy with lowest possible dose. **Oxcarbamazepine**, the prodrug of CBZ appears to have similar risk profile; however, enough data is not available at present [5]. Second line drugs, lamotrigine and baclofen have shown promise in the management of TGN [6, 7]; the former has been found to be more efficacious than CBZ. Although a category C drug (USFDA), **Lamotrigine** has been reported to be safe in pregnancy, in recent studies [8, 9]. Therefore, it can be a useful alternative to CBZ in pregnant patients. Occurrence of skin rashes in some of the patients is a major concern, which can prevented by slow titration of the dose. **Baclofen** is a useful second-line drug in the treatment of TGN and the action is very much similar to that of CBZ [10]. There are reports of uneventful fetal outcome after intrathecal use for multiple sclerosis during pregnancy [11]. Nevertheless, reports of neonatal baclofen withdrawal after prenatal exposure can be a major deterrent to its use in pregnancy [12, 13]. Apart from the main stream therapies, drugs like gabapentin, pregabalin, topiramate and levetiracetam have been tried as monotherapy or as adjuvants in TGN. Gabapentin has not been associated with major fetal malformations, but incidences of low birth weight and preterm delivery has been reported [14]. **Pregabalin** has been associated with fetal malformations in rat model [15]; no human study carried out to determine its safety in pregnancy. **Topiramate** is absolutely contraindicated in pregnancy as it is associated with cleft lip and palate in fetus [16]. **Levetiracetam**, a newer AED and recently been used as monotherapy or add-on drug in TGN with good success. Enough literature suggested it as one of the safest drug during pregnancy [17]. However, further studies are needed to prove its efficacy in TGN. There has been a growing interest about the use of **botulinum neurotoxin A (BoNT-A)** and the available evidence is encouraging [18, 19]. USFDA recommends it to be administered in pregnancy only if the benefit outweigh the potential risk to the fetus. In a survey of treating physicians who routinely used BoNT-A, there was no report of quantitative association of its injection with any adverse outcome of pregnancy including miscarriage or fetal malformation [20].

It is worth mentioning that the risk of fetal adverse effect is maximum during the phase of organogenesis, that is, between 4 and 10 weeks of gestation. After 10 weeks, the effects are mainly defective organogenesis and intrauterine growth retardation of fetus [21]. Hence, it is wise not to prescribe drugs like CBZ and other potential teratogenic agents during the first few weeks of pregnancy. Alternatively, medications such as lamotrigine, levetiracetam or BoNT-A therapy may be considered, or non-pharmacologic modalities has to be planned.

Interventional Therapy

Interventional pain relieving procedures are probably the best way forward in pregnant women when conventional drugs are contraindicated or second-line drugs are ineffective. There are several interventions available which can be broadly classified in to open surgical and percutaneous interventions. Surgical procedures like **microvascular decompression (MVD)** is relatively contraindicated during pregnancy in view of the invasiveness of the procedure and the need of general anesthesia [22].

Percutaneous interventions are less invasive and can be done under local anesthesia in awake state. Gasserian ganglion rhizotomy is the commonest percutaneous procedure for TGN. It can be achieved either by radio frequency ablation or chemical neurolysis or by balloon micro-compression [23]. **Radio-frequency ablation** (RFA) of Gasserian ganglion is one of the most popular intervention [24]. However, there are few concerns, regarding performing these procedures in pregnancy. The primary concern is the harmful effect of radiation on the fetus as this procedure is done under fluoroscopic guidance. Evidently, the risk of radiation injury to the fetus depends on the stage of fetal development and the magnitude of radiation. The fetus is most sensitive to the radiation effect during the period of organogenesis and in the early fetal period. Moreover, any radiation dose below 50 mGy is not associated with increased risk of developmental anomaly [25]. Hence, it is advisable to perform fluoroscopic-guided procedures preferably in the 2nd and 3rd trimester of pregnancy. In addition to that, all effort has to be directed towards reducing the radiation exposure by using intermittent fluoroscopy, low magnification, electronic collimation, and wrapping of the patient with lead shield [26]. Apart from the radiation effects, there are concerns of radio frequency ablation adversely affecting utero-placental circulation and labor precipitation. No prior data is available on RFA use in pregnancy, except a recently reported case by the author, where RFA was done successfully in a pregnant woman suffering from TGN [1]. Besides that there are reports of safe use of RFA in pregnancy for indications like intramural fibroid, ablation of cardiac conduction pathway in refractory arrhythmia [27, 28]. **Percutaneous glycerol rhizotomy** and **percutaneous balloon microcompression** are other two equally effective percutaneous interventions, which can also be performed, though currently no data available of their use in pregnant females.

Peripheral trigeminal nerve blocks though less effective than central ganglion level procedure, can be useful when the latter is unsuitable [29]. There is no risk of radiation exposure to the fetus, as it is done either by eliciting paresthesia or by using peripheral nerve simulator or under USG guidance [30, 31]. In pregnant woman, peripheral nerve blocks may be a credible options in controlling pain especially during the first trimester, when other procedures are relatively contraindicated.

Gamma knife radio surgery (GKRS) has been established as a non-invasive outpatient procedure for TGN [32]. It involves a high dose (70–80 Gy) focused radiation beam directed to the trigeminal root [33]. There are case reports mentioning minimal radiation exposure to fetus in pregnant women undergoing GKRS for cerebral malignancies [34]. However, it is too early to consider it as a treatment modality for TGN during pregnancy, especially when other relatively safer options are available.

Conclusion

Rare co-existence of TGN in pregnant woman and paucity of previous data may present a unique management challenge to the clinicians. It should be kept in mind that the treatment options available to treat TGN are not 100% safe in pregnancy. However, it could be an overstatement, and each treatment modality has to be weighed in terms of risk-benefit ratio. If a woman suffering from TGN plans for pregnancy, she has to be counselled about the pros and cons of all treatment modalities available, and an informed decision might be undertaken based on the available resources and expertise. It is better to withhold all teratogenic medications including carbamazepine once the diagnosis of pregnancy is established, and it has to be substituted with relatively safer second-line medications. If medical management fails to achieve good pain relief, minimally invasive percutaneous procedures should be considered. Nonetheless, it is safe to avoid procedures requiring fluoroscopy in the first trimester when the fetus is most vulnerable to the radiation injury.

References

1. Swain BP, Vidhya S, Jadon A, Chandra KN, Kumar S. Trigeminal neuralgia in pregnancy: a management challenge. Pain Pract. 2018;18:368–73.
2. FDA pregnancy risk information: an update. Available from: https://www.drugs.com/pregnancy-categories.html.

3. Australian Department of Health. Therapeutic Goods Administration. Prescribing medicines in pregnancy database. Available from: http://www.tga.gov.au/hp/medicines-pregnancy.htm. Accessed Apr 24, 2018.
4. Vajda FJE, O'Brien TJ, Graham J, Lander CM, Eadie MJ. Is carbamazepine a human teratogen? J Clin Neurosci. 2015;23:34–7.
5. Montouris G. Safety of the newer antiepileptic drug oxcarbazepine during pregnancy. Curr Med Res Opin. 2005;21:693–701.
6. Shaikh S, Yaacob HB, Abd Rahman RB. Lamotrigine for trigeminal neuralgia: efficacy and safety in comparison with carbamazepine. J Chin Med Assoc. 2011;74:243–9.
7. Fromm GH, Terrence CF, Chattha AS. Baclofen in the treatment of trigeminal neuralgia: double-blind study and long-term follow-up. Ann Neurol. 1984;15:240–4.
8. Dolk H, Wang H, Loane M, Morris J, Garne E, Addor MC, et al. Lamotrigine use in pregnancy and risk of orofacial cleft and other congenital anomalies. Neurology. 2016;86:1716–25.
9. Wise J. Study finds lamotrigine to be safe during pregnancy. BMJ. 2017;359:j4827.
10. Parmar BS, Shah KH, Gandhi IC. Baclofen in trigeminal neuralgia—a clinical trial. Indian J Dent Res. 1989:109–13.
11. Dalton CM, Keenan E, Jarrett L, Buckley L, Stevenson VL. The safety of baclofen in pregnancy: intrathecal therapy in multiple sclerosis. Mult Scler. 2008;14:571–2.
12. Freeman EH, Delaney RM. Neonatal baclofen withdrawal: a case report of an infant presenting with severe feeding difficulties. J Pediatr Nurs. 2016;31:346–9.
13. Baclofen and pregnancy: birth defects and withdrawal symptoms. Prescrire Int. 2015; 24:214.
14. Fujii H, Goel A, Bernard N, et al. Pregnancy outcomes following gabapentin use: results of a prospective comparative cohort study. Neurology. 2013;80:1565–70.
15. Hill DS, Wlodarczyk BJ, Palacios AM, Finnell RH. Teratogenic effects of antiepileptic drugs. Expert Rev Neurother. 2010;10:943–59.
16. Margulis AV, Mitchell AA, Gilboa SM, Werler MM, Mittleman MA, Glynn RJ, Hernandez-Diaz S, National Birth Defects Prevention Study. Use of topiramate in pregnancy and risk of oral clefts. Am J Obstet Gynecol. 2012;207:405.e1–7.
17. Koubeissi M. Levetiracetam: more evidence of safety in pregnancy. Epilepsy Currents. 2013;13:279–81.
18. Morra ME, Elgebaly A, Elmaraezy A, Khalil AM, Altibi AM, Vu TL, et al. Therapeutic efficacy and safety of Botulinum Toxin A therapy in trigeminal neuralgia: a systematic review and meta-analysis of randomized controlled trials. J Headache Pain. 2016;17:63.
19. Wu CJ, Lian YJ, Zheng YK, Zhang HF, Chen Y, Xie NC, et al. Botulinum toxin type A for the treatment of trigeminal neuralgia: results from a randomized, double-blind, placebo controlled trial. Cephalalgia. 2012;32:443–50.
20. Morgan JC, Iyer SS, Moser ET, Singer C, Sethi KD. Botulinum toxin A during pregnancy: a survey of treating physicians. J Neurol Neurosurg Psychiatry. 2006;77:117–9.
21. Gilbert-Barness E. Teratogenic causes of malformations. Ann Clin Lab Sci Spring. 2010;40:99–114.
22. Al-Quliti KW. Update on neuropathic pain treatment for trigeminal neuralgia: the pharmacological and surgical options. Neurosciences. 2015;20:107–14.
23. Pollock BE. Surgical management of medically refractory trigeminal neuralgia. Curr Neurol Neurosci Rep. 2012;12:125–31.
24. Lopez BC, Hamlyn PJ, Zakrzewska JM. Systematic review of ablative neurosurgical techniques for the treatment of trigeminal neuralgia. Neurosurgery. 2004;54:973–82.
25. American College of Radiology. ACR-SPR practice parameter for imaging pregnant or potentially pregnant adolescents and women with ionizing radiation. Available from: http://www.acr.org/media/ACR/Documents/PGTS/guidelines/Pregnant_Patients.pdf.
26. Shaw P, Duncan A, Vouyouka A, Ozsvath K. Radiation exposure and pregnancy. J Vasc Surg. 2011;53:28S–34S.
27. Berman JM, Puscheck EE, Diamond MP. Full term vaginal live birth after laparoscopic radiofrequency ablation of a large, symptomatic intramural fibroid: A case report. J Reprod Med. 2012;57:159–63.

28. Kanjwal Y, Kosinski D, Kani M, Thomas W, Grubb B. Successful radiofrequency catheter ablation of left lateral accessory pathway using transseptal approach during pregnancy. J Interv Card Electrophysiol. 2005;13:239–42.
29. Peters G, Nurmikko TJ. Peripheral and gasserian ganglion-level procedures for the treatment of trigeminal neuralgia. Clin J Pain. 2002;18:28–34.
30. Kumar N, Shashni S, Singh R, Jain A. Mandibular nerve block for peri-operative pain relief using a peripheral nerve stimulator. Anaesthesia. 2012;67:77–8.
31. Nader A, Schittek H, Kendall MC. Lateral pterygoid muscle and maxillary artery are key anatomical landmarks for ultrasound-guided trigeminal nerve block. Anesthesiology. 2013;118:957.
32. Gorgulho AA, De Salles AA. Impact of radiosurgery on the surgical treatment of trigeminal neuralgia. Surg Neurol. 2006;66:350–6.
33. Kondziolka D, Lunsford LD, Flickinger JC. Stereotactic radiosurgery for the treatment of trigeminal neuralgia. Clin J Pain. 2002;18:42–7.
34. Yu C, Jozsef G, Apuzzo ML, MacPherson DM, Petrovich Z. Fetal radiation doses for model C gamma knife radiosurgery. Neurosurgery. 2003;52:687–93.

Trigemino-Cardiac Reflex and Trigeminal Neuralgia

Varun Jain and Gyaninder Pal Singh

Key Points

- Trigemino-cardiac reflex (TCR) is one of the most powerful autonomic response of the human body commonly presents with sudden severe bradycardia and hypotension
- Surgical interventions for trigeminal neuralgia such as microvascular decompression, percutaneous radiofrequency thermocoagulation, glycerol rhizolysis, and balloon compression are known to be associated with TCR
- Removal of the triggering factor usually abolishes TCR, though in few cases it may require use of drugs, and even, cardiac life support in refractory conditions

Introduction

Depressor response on heart due to stimulation of sensory branches of trigeminal nerve have been known since a long time. However, a formal interest in trigemino-cardiac reflex (TCR) grew after its introduction to neurosurgery in 1999 [1]. TCR is one of the strongest autonomic response and shows the complex relationship between brain and heart. There is no formal definition for the reflex; the widely accepted definition suggests TCR as a sudden fall in heart rate and mean blood pressure (BP) by 20% or more during surgical manipulation of structures innervated by the trigeminal nerve [2]. A definition to encompass other clinical manifestation of efferent vagal nerve suggests that trigemino-vagal reflex is an autonomic manifestation (e.g. change in breathing pattern and gastrointestinal motility) with or without

V. Jain · G. P. Singh (✉)
Department of Neuroanaesthesiology and Critical Care, All India Institute of Medical Sciences (AIIMS), New Delhi, India

G. P. Rath (ed.), *Handbook of Trigeminal Neuralgia*,
https://doi.org/10.1007/978-981-13-2333-1_30

change in heart rate or BP, coinciding with the stimulation of trigeminal nerve. Because bradycardia can be observed during operative procedures due to several reasons, a cause-effect relationship must be established to label a bradycardic episode as TCR. The cause–effect relationship can be established if TCR appears promptly on application of stimulus within 5 s (plausibility); stimulus cessation brings back the cardiovascular changes to baseline (reversibility); reapplication of similar stimulus leads to same hemodynamic changes (repetition); and trigeminal nerve block or use of anticholinergics or lower intensity stimulus does not lead to a repeat response (prevention) [2].

Etiopathogenesis of TCR

Anatomic Pathway: TCR is a brainstem reflex and has been found to be present even in decerebated animals in experimental studies [3]. Afferent fibers are branches of trigeminal nerves which relay the signals via Gasserian ganglion (GG) to the sensory portion of trigeminal nucleus located in the brainstem. From there short internuncial fibers (SIF) of reticular formation transfers the signal to the vagus nerve nucleus. Vagus nerve carries the information to the myocardium (Fig. 1). There is a difference in the way signals are relayed to depressor fibers of myocardium depending on where the trigeminal nerve is stimulated. If the stimulation is of peripheral nerve endings proximal to reaching the GG, it is called ***Peripheral TCR***, and when stimulation is of the intracranial portion of the trigeminal nerve after the GG, it is called ***Central TCR***. In Central TCR, the impulses are not relayed via the main sensory nucleus of trigeminal nerve but are conducted from GG to the SIF via nucleus tractus solitarius and lateral parabrachial nucleus.

Ophthalmocardiac reflex (OCR), maxillomandibulo-cardiac reflex, and diving reflex are various subtypes of peripheral TCR. In OCR, long and short ciliary nerves are stimulated to conduct impulses via ciliary ganglion to the GG. In Diving reflex, the anterior ethmoidal nerves of nasal mucosa are stimulated. Impulses further to

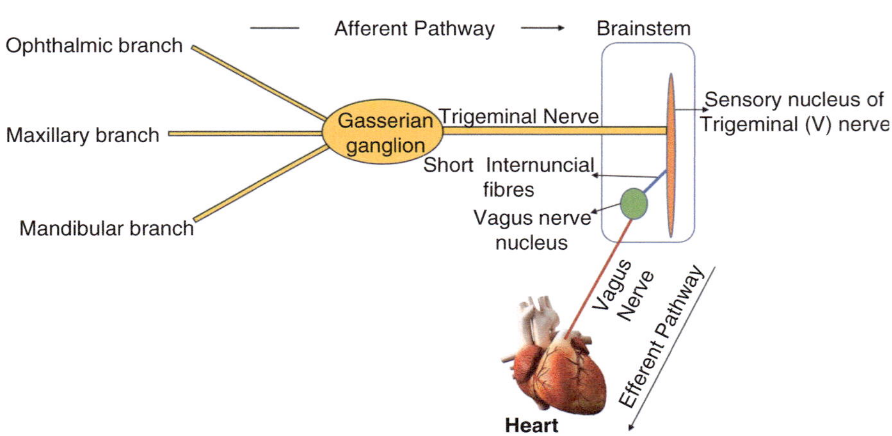

Fig. 1 Trigemino-cardiac reflex pathway

Table 1 Clinical scenarios associated with TCR

• Ophthalmic Surgery [20]—strabismus correction, foreign bodies removal, cataract surgeries, enucleation, iridectomy, acute glaucoma
• Cranio-facial surgeries—Le-fort I osteotomies, zygomatic arc fracture repair
• Cerebellopontine angle tumors surgery [1]
• Trigeminal neuralgia treatment [9] e.g. microvascular decompression (Janetta procedure), balloon rhizotomy
• Transsphenoidal surgeries for invasive pituitary macroadenomas [21]
• Posterior circulation aneurysm clipping surgery
• Chronic subdural hematoma evacuation
• Neurointerventional procedures—Glue embolization of juvenile nasopharyngeal angiofibroma [22]

Table 2 Peri-procedural risk factors for increased occurrence of trigeminocardiac reflex [23]

• Hypoxemia
• Hypercarbia
• Light plane of anesthesia
• Young age (high vagal tone)
• Stronger and longer duration of stimulus
• Drugs such as opioids, beta-blockers, calcium channel blockers

GG are transmitted via spinal trigeminal nucleus, pars caudalis and Kölliker-Fuse nucleus to SIF [4]. Diving reflex is frequently associated with bradycardia and hypertension [4].

TCR also represents a subtype of '**Oxygen-Conserving Reflex**' phenomenon [5]. Within seconds of the activation of this reflex, there is an increase in cerebral blood flow due to differentiated activation of sympathetic system, without any increase in oxygen or glucose demand by the brain. Therefore, there is primary cerebrovascular vasodilatation and increase oxygen reserve for the brain despite occurrence of hypotension and apnea. The associated bradycardia also causes reduction of oxygen consumption by the heart and thus preserves body oxygen. Clear pathway for this reflex has not been defined. However, the impulses are supposed to travel from rostral ventrolateral medulla oblongata to upper brainstem and thalamus and few fibers are connected to cerebral cortex. This cortical center leads to reflex cerebral vasodilatation, a phenomenon which is unique among such autonomic reflexes.

Causes of TCR: There are various surgical and neurointerventional procedures when TCR has been reported (Table 1) [6]. Apart from these procedures, there are certain predisposing factors which increase the risk of a patient to develop TCR (Table 2).

Clinical Manifestation

The most consistent clinical manifestation of TCR is bradycardia. A sudden fall in heart rate by 38–46% with return to baseline values after removing the surgical stimulus during various neurosurgical procedures, has been described. Bradycardia may

Table 3 Variants of TCR and their clinical manifestations

Trigger	Heart rate	Blood pressure	Apnea/gastric hypermotility
1. Stimulation of areas innervated by ophthalmic maxillary & mandibular branches ***(Peripheral TCR)***	Decrease	Decrease or normal (increase in DR)	Present
2. Stimulation of Gasserian ganglion ***(Ganglionic TCR)***	Decrease or increase	Decrease or increase	Present
3. Stimulation of intracranial part of trigeminal nerve proximal to Gasserian ganglion ***(Central TCR)***	Decrease	Decrease	Present

TCR Trigeminocardiac reflex, *DR* Diving reflex

advance to asystole or there can be sudden asystole without any prior warning bradycardia. The period of asystole usually lasts for 30–70 s with return of normal heart rate over next 90–180 s following release of inflicting stimuli [1]. Tachycardia is an unusual manifestation of TCR, and can occur in procedures involved in direct stimulation of GG [2]. Besides these, persistent dysrhythmia such as premature atrial contractions [7], could be a sole manifestation of TCR. Changes in BP is another frequent clinical manifestation. Hypotension is commonly observed in central TCR, whereas peripheral TCR is usually associated with normotension. Hypotension is sudden, with a fall in mean arterial BP by 48–54% from baseline. During diving reflex, bradycardia is associated with hypertension due to peripheral vasoconstriction [8]. Direct stimulation of GG may also lead to hypertensive response.

Apnea is another consistent finding in TCR. The apneic response is missed during intraoperative period, as it occurs while the patient is sedated and mechanically ventilated. Gastric hypermotility is also observed as a part of the TCR response. Various variants of TCR and their manifestations are given in Table 3.

TCR During Interventional Pain Management for TGN

Incidence of TCR during treatment of TGN is unclear. Schaller B [9] reported occurrence of TCR in patients of TGN undergoing ***Microvascular Decompression (MVD)***. Five out of 28 patients operated over a period of 8 years in this study had TCR. In all these patient, general anesthesia was maintained with isoflurane, along with fentanyl and atracurium. Teflon graft was placed between the impinging blood vessel and the root entry zone (REZ) of trigeminal nerve. A temporal association was found between patients on calcium channel blockers and TCR; however, it was not so in patients receiving other medications such as beta-blockers and carbamazepine. One of the five patients who suffered TCR had asystole, but heart rate returned back to baseline values after the surgical stimulus was withdrawn. It has been observed that abrupt and sudden traction (triggering factor; mechanical) causes TCR more than the smooth and gentle traction. Use of atropine prevented further development of TCR response during the course of surgery. Authors suggested to monitor direct arterial BP for 24 h during postoperative period as the occurrence of TCR is not predictable.

Meng and colleagues [10] examined the effect of ***Percutaneous Radiofrequency Thermocoagulation*** in the patients with primary TGN. They observed occurrence of bradycardia and hypertension in 6 out of total 48 patients, at the time of puncture of foramen ovale. This response rapidly reverted back to baseline values on interruption of surgical maneuver. However, the pressor response (e.g. tachycardia and hypertension) was observed consistently in all patients, at the time of electrical stimulation and thermocoagulation (triggering factors). The magnitude of pressure response and temperature of radiofrequency thermocoagulation were positively correlated when the temperature setting was less than 75 °C. This correlation became negative when temperature was increased to more than 75 °C. Pressor manifestation of TCR during radiofrequency thermo-ablation suggests different transduction mechanism and pathway during high and low heat is responsible for such an effect [11]. Also, this pressor response cannot be abolished by using increasing doses of analgesics [10, 12] but they can be abolished by injection of lidocaine into the Meckel's cave before compression of the ganglion [10].

Percutaneous Retrogasserian Glycerol Rhizolysis (PRGR) under general anesthesia has been shown to cause severe bradycardia [13]. This occurred sometime after the entry of needle into the trigeminal cistern, and it was hypothesized that CSF drainage causing traction of dura (mechanical trigger) in the middle cranial fossa innervated by meningeal branch of maxillary nerve, or use of dye or glycerol (chemical trigger), or use of radiofrequency (electrical trigger) led to occurrence of TCR. The reflex responded to injection of glycopyrrolate, in these patients. Similarly, Rath et al. [14] reported cardio-respiratory arrest with unconsciousness, during glycerol injection (chemical trigger) in trigeminal cistern for PRGR. During this episode, the patient responded to injection of atropine. The procedure was abandoned and rescheduled a week later with atropine premedication. However, severe bradycardia was still encountered, intraprocedurally, requiring repeated injections of intravenous atropine.

Mullan and colleagues [15] observed significant transient bradycardia while engaging the needle into the foramen ovale and during distension of the balloon (mechanical trigger) during ***Percutaneous Balloon Compression*** to treat TGN. Once the nerve was compressed adequately, bradycardia did not recur with further compressions. Because of the co-activation of sympathetic and parasympathetic nervous system during balloon micro-compression, TCR manifests as bradycardia, tachycardia or arrhythmia with hypo or hypertension. Chen et al. [16] observed the effect of atropine (0.01 mg/kg) with labetalol (0.05 mg/kg) given 3 min prior to balloon compression. Both the agents were able to reduce the frequency of bradycardia but neither of them could abolish the TCR response completely. Labetalol was more effective in preventing the post-compression tachycardia.

Treatment of TCR

A careful, vigilant, and continuous hemodynamic monitoring for atleast first 24 h after the procedure is prudent to be warned about the occurrence of TCR. Removal of triggering factor often abolishes the reflex, and brings back the heart rate and BP to normal. Predisposing risk factors such as hypercarbia, hypoxia, light plane of anesthesia, and acidosis must be corrected to prevent aggravation of TCR. Anticholinergics may be needed in certain cases with severe bradycardia which does not revert back to normal after withdrawing the stimulus. Intramuscular anticholinergics are not effective in preventing TCR, and therefore prophylactic administration is not advocated especially in cases where central TCR is expected [6, 14]. Adrenaline may be needed in rare scenarios suggesting that TCR can also occur due to loss of sympathetic tone rather than increased vagal tone [4]. Occasionally, vasopressors and immediate cardiac life support may be needed in case of intractable cardiac events [4, 6]. Peripheral nerve blockade which constitutes the afferent limb of the TCR has been shown to be effective in preventing peripheral TCR [4].

Future Research Direction

Intraoperative TCR during the excision of vestibular schwannoma and pituitary adenoma has been observed to be associated with worse functional outcome with postoperative ipsilateral tinnitus, hearing loss, or increased pituitary hormonal insufficiency [17, 18]. However, it is unclear, whether occurrence of TCR during treatment of TGN is associated with similar adverse outcomes. Similarly, a newer terminology called 'chronic TCR' has emerged in recent years to explain the vague autonomic symptoms (especially nausea and vomiting) days, months or years after the insult to peripheral trigeminal nerve [19]. Since, TGN is a long-standing suffering often requiring multimodal treatment strategy, whether some cases are a reflection of this 'chronic TCR' needs to be dealt with in future.

Conclusion

The treatment of TGN may be associated with TCR. The presentation of TCR is varied and is a manifestation of simultaneous stimulation of both sympathetic and parasympathetic autonomic nervous system. Although, the cardiovascular manifestations are usually benign and revert back on interruption of the stimulus, awareness, high degree of suspicion, and close observation are important to identify the condition so as to prevent any untoward event. The physicians and surgeons treating such patients should be vigilant and prepared to manage any eventuality including the need for acute cardiac life support.

References

1. Schaller B, Probst R, Strebel S, Gratzl O. Trigeminocardiac reflex during surgery in the cerebellopontine angle. J Neurosurg. 1999;90:215–20.

2. Meuwly C, Golanov E, Chowdhury T, Erne P, Schaller B. Trigeminal cardiac reflex: new thinking model about the definition based on a literature review. Medicine (Baltimore). 2015;94:e484.
3. Kumada M, Dampney RA, Reis DJ. The trigeminal depressor response: a novel vasodepressor response originating from the trigeminal system. Brain Res. 1977;119:305–26.
4. Abdulazim A, Stienen MN, Sadr-Eshkevari P, Prochnow N, Sandu N, Bohluli B, et al. Trigeminocardiac reflex in neurosurgery—current knowledge and prospects. In: Explicative Cases of Controversial Issues in Neurosurgery. InTech; 2012.
5. Sandu N, Spiriev T, Lemaitre F, Filis A, Schaller B, Trigemino-Cardiac-Reflex-Examination-Group (T.C.R.E.G.). New molecular knowledge towards the trigemino-cardiac reflex as a cerebral oxygen-conserving reflex. Sci World J. 2010;10:811–7.
6. Schaller B, Cornelius JF, Prabhakar H, Koerbel A, Gnanalingham K, Sandu N, et al. The trigemino-cardiac reflex. J Neurosurg Anesthesiol. 2009;21:187–95.
7. Rath GP, Sharma VB, Dube SK. Persistent premature atrial contraction as the sole presentation of trigeminocardiac reflex during radiofrequency thermocoagulation. J Neurosurg Anesthesiol. 2017;29:187–8.
8. Panneton WM. The mammalian diving response: an enigmatic reflex to preserve life? Physiology (Bethesda). 2013;28:284–97.
9. Schaller B. Trigemino-cardiac reflex during microvascular trigeminal decompression in cases of trigeminal neuralgia. J Neurosurg Anesthesiol. 2005;17:45–8.
10. Meng Q, Zhang W, Yang Y, Zhou M, Li X. Cardiovascular responses during percutaneous radiofrequency thermocoagulation therapy in primary trigeminal neuralgia. J Neurosurg Anesthesiol. 2008;20:131–5.
11. Schaller B, Sandu N, Filis A, Buchfelder M, Trigemino-Cardiac-Reflex-Examination-Group. Cardiovascular responses during percutaneous radiofrequency thermocoagulation therapy in primary trigeminal neuralgia: an explanation of the trigeminocardiac reflex? J Neurosurg Anesthesiol. 2008;20:270.
12. Sweet WH, Poletti CE, Roberts JT. Dangerous rises in blood pressure upon heating of trigeminal rootlets; increased bleeding times in patients with trigeminal neuralgia. Neurosurgery. 1985;17:843–4.
13. Chowdhury T, Cappellani RB, Schaller B, for Trigeminocardiac Reflex Examination Group (TCREG). Retrogasserian glycerol rhizolysis: first description of occurrence trigeminocardiac reflex. J Neurosurg Anesthesiol. 2014;26:86–7.
14. Rath GP, Dash HH, Prabhakar H, Pandia MP. Cardiorespiratory arrest during trigeminal rhizolysis. Anaesthesia. 2007;62:971–2.
15. Mullan S, Lichtor T. Percutaneous microcompression of the trigeminal ganglion for trigeminal neuralgia. J Neurosurg. 1983;59:1007–12.
16. Chen CY, Luo CF, Hsu YC, Chen JF, Day YJ. Comparison of the effects of atropine and labetalol on trigeminocardiac reflex-induced hemodynamic alterations during percutaneous microballoon compression of the trigeminal ganglion. Acta Anaesthesiol Taiwanica. 2012;50:153–8.
17. Gharabaghi A, Koerbel A, Samii A, Kaminsky J, von Goesseln H, Tatagiba M, et al. The impact of hypotension due to the trigeminocardiac reflex on auditory function in vestibular schwannoma surgery. J Neurosurg. 2006;104:369–75.
18. Chowdhury T, Nöthen C, Filis A, Sandu N, Buchfelder M, Schaller B. Functional outcome changes in surgery for pituitary adenomas after intraoperative occurrence of the trigeminocardiac reflex: first description in a retrospective observational study. Medicine (Baltimore). 2015;94:e1463.
19. Chowdhury T, Schaller B. Chronic trigemino-cardiac reflex: an underestimated truth. Front Neurol. 2017;8:22.
20. Alexander JP. Reflex disturbances of cardiac rhythm during ophthalmic surgery. Br J Ophthalmol. 1975;59:518–24.
21. Schaller B. Trigemino-cardiac reflex during transsphenoidal surgery for pituitary adenomas. Clin Neurol Neurosurg. 2005;107:468–74.

22. Puri AS, Thiex R, Zarzour H, Rahbar R, Orbach DB. Trigeminocardiac reflex in a child during pre-Onyx DMSO injection for juvenile nasopharyngeal angiofibroma embolization. A case report. Interv Neuroradiol. 2011;17:13–6.
23. Meuwly C, Chowdhury T, Sandu N, Reck M, Erne P, Schaller B. Anesthetic influence on occurrence and treatment of the trigemino-cardiac reflex: a systematic literature review. Medicine (Baltimore). 2015;94:e807.

Therapeutic Outcome and Future Scopes in the Management of Trigeminal Neuralgia

W. Umamaheshwara Rao and Muralidhar Joshi

Key Points

- Treatment for trigeminal neuralgia (TGN) includes several modalities, each with variable efficacy or notable adverse effects
- Novel therapeutic options, like BIB074 which are in advanced clinical testing, may be available very soon
- Botulinum neurotoxin type A is an additional add-on treatment option for TGN patients without major systemic side-effects
- Emerging non-drug medical therapy encompasses non-invasive neuromodulation techniques

Introduction

Trigeminal neuralgia (TGN) is an elusive medical condition with debilitating consequences. Treatment options for TGN have evolved and improved over the years; however, many existing drugs and percutaneous procedures have variable efficacy and recurrence is possible in many patients. Many new molecules acting on novel pain targets are being studied, which are in pre-clinical, or early clinical development phases. Various surgical therapies have been tried for the management of drug-resistant TGN. Among them, microvascular decompression (MVD) is performed to address the primary problem of aberrant vascular loops impinging on the trigeminal

W. Umamaheshwara Rao
Anaesthesiologist and Interventional Pain Specialist, Virinchi Hospitals, Hyderabad, Telangana, India

M. Joshi (✉)
Pain Management Centre, Virinchi Hospitals, Hyderabad, Telangana, India

G. P. Rath (ed.), *Handbook of Trigeminal Neuralgia*,
https://doi.org/10.1007/978-981-13-2333-1_31

nerve. On the other hand, percutaneous destructive procedures aim at reducing the overall sensory input from the trigeminal ganglion.

Medical Management and Outcome

Current Pharmocotherapy

Phenytoin was the first therapeutic drug used for TGN with significant positive effects [1]. Current recommendations are to start carbamazepine (CBZ) and oxcarbazepine (OXC) as first-line therapy for TGN [2]. Three randomized controlled trials (RCTs) comparing OXC to CBZ in TGN patients reported a reduction in the frequency and intensity of attacks; and assessment for pain was comparable after both CBZ and OXC, with more than 80% of patients reporting 'very good' response to these drugs [3–5]. Several other drugs have been used such as baclofen, lamotrigine, pimozide and tocainide [6]. Lamotrigine, when administered along with CBZ or phenytoin, has been found to be more effective than placebo [7, 8]. In patients who have already undergone surgery, or are taking concurrent medications, tizanidine has also been found to be better than placebo, but its effect decays within one to three months [9]. Topical ophthalmic anesthesia is unlikely to be very effective as an analgesic measure in patients with TGN. It is unclear whether polytherapy is superior to monotherapy [10]. There is also insufficient evidence regarding the efficacy of intravenous (IV) fosphenytoin or other IV medications for the treatment of acute exacerbations of TGN.

Emerging Medical Therapy

It is well-known that TGN can be very difficult to treat and may recur even after neurosurgical intervention. A recent article suggests that oral gabapentin combined with trigger site injections of ropivacaine improves pain-control and quality of life [11]. Pregabalin has also been seen to be effective in at 1-year follow-up of TGN patients. Hu et al. reviewed the use of botulinum neurotoxin type A (BoNT-A) injections in TGN. They found good response in 70–100% of patients, with diminished pain intensity by 60–80% without major adverse events [12]. These results are in agreement with the study by Cruccu and Truini, which also found evidence supporting BoNT-A injections in drug-refractory TGN patients, before surgery, or in those unwilling to undergo surgery [13]. Although BoNT represents a promising modality of treatment for TGN with favourable risk-to-benefit ratio, further well-designed RCTs are needed to define the optimal dose, duration of therapeutic efficacy, side effects, and the time and indications for repeat injection. Acute painful crisis is a complicated scenario; ropivacaine injected into the trigger area, lignocaine 8% spray, and IV infusion of fosphenytoin can provide temporary pain relief [11].

Selective sodium channels like $Na_v1.7$, have been linked to neuropathic pain, especially painful sensory neuropathies and TGN. Vixotrigine, a small novel molecule, was earlier suggested to be a selective peripheral $Na_v1.7$ blocker. It has now been re-defined as a non-selective voltage-gated sodium channel blocker and is undergoing phase III clinical trial for its use in TGN. Other novel compounds are in preclinical or early clinical phase of development for neuropathic pain; but, there is emerging evidence of the potential clinical utility of $Na_v1.7$ antagonists and angiotensin type II inhibitors in neuropathic pain [14].

Surgical Interventions and Outcome

Surgical options are reserved for cases refractory to medical management or when side effects of medications exceed risks and drawbacks of surgery. Surgical treatments can be broadly classified as (a) peripheral procedures, (b) Gasserian ganglion procedures, and (c) posterior fossa procedures.

Peripheral Procedures

These are destructive procedures aimed at delivering treatment at the level of trigger point. Interventions includes: (1) Peripheral neurectomy, (2) Cryotherapy, (3) Injection of substances such as streptomycin, lignocaine, and bupivacaine, (4) Laser therapy and (5) Radiofrequency (RF) thermocoagulation/lesioning.

Peripheral Nerve Blocks (Neurectomy)

The role of nerve blocks is to provide pain relief when pharmacological management is unsuccessful, or it is used as an adjunct to allow reduction in dose of drugs. Individual divisions of the fifth nerve may be blocked with local anesthetic (LA) agents, where they leave the skull and enter the face and mouth. In addition to their diagnostic value, it is not uncommon for these blocks to break a cycle of pain. Subsequently, pain relief may be obtained for much longer than duration of action of the LA. There could be a high rate of recurrence and late deafferentation pain, hence, caution needs to be exercised [15]. Danish investigators found that in patients who underwent neurectomy, pain-recurrence was seen in 78% of patients within 7 years; with first recurrence within a month in 50% of patients. Moreover, neurectomy (as well as alcohol block) leads to less efficacious results compared to RF lesioning [16].

Cryotherapy

Cryotherapy involves ablation of a peripheral branch of the trigeminal nerve by direct application of a probe with tip temperatures ranging between −50 °C and −70 °C. A standard protocol for cryotherapy is 3-cycles of 2-min freezing followed by a 5-min thaw. This procedure requires sedation or general anesthesia (GA) [15]. Although cryotherapy is tolerated well by the patients, results are modest. Of 145 patients went through 1 to 11 sessions of cryotherapy, pain relief lasted less than 6 months in 50%, and at 1 year, only 27% patients were pain-free. Although improvement in individual nerves with regard to pain was good, cryosurgery seems to be inferior to procedures aimed at the trigeminal ganglion, or the trigeminal root [17].

Laser Therapy

Low-level laser therapy (LLLT) uses a single wavelength light source, and works on the principle that irradiation with monochromatic light may affect cell function. This technique involves irradiation of the region of interest followed by laser puncture of predetermined points along the course of the nerve. The treatment is first given intra-orally for a period of 1–2 min, then extra-orally, to ensure laser puncture of the ‘bio-active points’ along the nerve path. Treatment duration is 10 min per day for 10–12 days. Stefanoff found that pain-free periods achieved with laser procedures were longer than those achieved with other methods [18].

Samosiuk and colleagues divided 137 patients with typical TGN into four groups. Thirty patients (G1) received extremely high frequency puncture (EHF) therapy, 30 patients were exposed to laser (G2), 67 patients were treated with combination of laser and EHF-puncture (G3), and 10 patients were in control group. All the patients were given CBZ. Best results were obtained from G3 in which 31% of patients could be withdrawn from CBZ, and in the rest of them in the group, drug-dose could be reduced by 50–70% [19].

Gasserian Ganglion Procedures

These procedures are popular interventions done in most patients under sedation or GA by inserting a needle into the Gasserian ganglion through the foramen ovale (FO). The needle position is checked by imaging, and then, several types of procedures such as percutaneous radiofrequency thermocoagulation (RFT), percutaneous retrogasserian glycerol rhizolysis (PRGR) and percutaneous balloon compression of the trigeminal nerve (PBC) are carried out.

Percutaneous Radiofrequency Thermocoagulation (RFT)

RF lesions are done at the Gasserian ganglion after an electrode is inserted through the FO under fluoroscopic control. The nerve can be coagulated by using temperatures of 60–80 °C for 60–90 s, which causes selective destruction of small pain fibres. Pain may recur in 20% of patients within 15 years. Scrivani et al. in a retrospective study of 215 patients, reported immediate pain relief in majority of patients (92%). The pain recurred in 27% patients at a mean follow-up of 32 months [20].

Percutaneous Retrogasserian Glycerol Rhizolysis (PRGR)

This procedure is common in the elderly. Pain may recur in 50% of patients within 3–4 years of blockade. Although pain relief is usually immediate after PRGR; it may take up to 7 days for the effect to come in some patients. Hakansson [21] reported initial pain relief in more than 80% of patients, however, the long-term results were variable. At 12 months, reported the recurrence rates varied from 10% to 53%. PRGR is generally well tolerated.

Alcohol Blocks: Peripheral and ganglionic alcohol blocks have lost popularity due to the variable outcomes and several reported adverse effects. Alcohol injections are administered directly into the nerve. The injections are intensely painful and are often followed by local edema [15]. After alcohol blocks the pain recurrence rate has been as high as 84% during a mean follow-up of 8 years. Nearly 50% of them had a recurrence within a month [16].

Percutaneous Balloon Compression (PBC) of the Trigeminal Nerve

The compression pressure from the balloon damages the nerve and blocks pain signals. It has been observed that 20% of the patients experience recurrence of pain within 3 years after the procedure. The balloon in Fogarty catheter is slowly inflated with approximately 0.5–1.0 mL of contrast agent until it expands to completely fill Meckel's cave, ensuring compression of the nerve. Total compression time may vary from 1 to 6 min. Kauzounias and colleagues studied the factors influencing the outcome after PBC for TGN [22]. There was no difference in the outcome based on the duration of compression of 60 s compared to longer time of compression. Patients with multiple sclerosis achieved similar benefit from the procedure as the patients with classic TGN [22]. Recurrence was reported in 6–14% cases in the first year. In one series, one-third of patients needed a repeat procedure during a mean follow-up of 4.3 years [23]. Lichtor and Mullan obtained slightly better results, recurrence was seen in only 20% of patients at 5 years follow-up, and 28% at 10 years [24].

Posterior Fossa Procedures

These procedures deliver treatment at the root entry zone (REZ), which is the cisternal part of the trigeminal nerve just as it enters the pons. These include microvascular decompression (MVD), partial sensory rhizotomy (PSR), and gamma knife radiosurgery (GKRS).

Microvascular Decompression

This procedure entails an open surgical approach to relieve compression of the trigeminal nerve at its root due to an aberrant vascular loop. Screening for neurovascular compression (NVC) should be done in patients with TGN, since NVC may affect patient selection, surgical planning, and outcomes. MVD is becoming increasingly popular in TGN, providing long-term pain relief. Unfortunately, all patients might not achieve good outcome following MVD [25]. The average duration of relief from pain following MVD is between 0.6 and 10 years [26]. After a period of 5 years, the percentage of pain free patients may range from 58% to 78% [27, 28]. In a study by Kondo, most patients (87–98%) experienced immediate pain relief following MVD. At 1–2 years, the incidence of complete pain relief was 75–80%, and after 8–10 years, this reduced to 58–64% [29].

Partial Sensory Rhizotomy

In this procedure, part of the trigeminal nerve at the base of the brain is severed. PSR is only carried out if no NVC is found on magnetic resonance imaging (MRI). PSR entails the division of the lateral part of the sensory root. In a 5-year follow up study, PSR was associated with a higher risk of postoperative complications than MVD [30].

Stereotactic Gamma Knife Radiosurgery

Gamma-knife radiosurgery (GKRS) is a valuable addition to the existing treatment options. It targets the nerve REZ with a high dose of radiation aimed at the root of the trigeminal nerve, destroying it. With GKRS, the pain recurs in 3–5 years in 50% of patients post-treatement [14]. Han et al. [31] studied the long-term outcome of GKRS for treatment of classical TGN in 62 patients. They observed the recurrence-free survival rate being 84.8%, 76.1%, 69.6%, 63.0%, and 45.8% at 1, 2, 3, 4, and 5 years after GKRS, respectively.

Outcome After Different Surgeries

All procedures are subject to technical or surgical failures, but most patients can expect to obtain complete pain relief for a brief period. In most instances, the more distal or peripheral is the procedure the earlier is the recurrence. On average, peripheral procedures provide less than a year of pain relief. Gasserian ganglion procedures and GKRS may provide a pain free period of 4 years in 50% patients, whereas MVD and partial sensory rhizotomy give a 70% pain relief for a duration of 10 years [28, 32]. Very few studies have measured secondary outcomes such as quality of life. Most studies found significant improvement in quality of life of patients who underwent MVD [33]. Patients who underwent Gasserian ganglion and posterior fossa surgeries were often able to discontinue all their medications.

Future Scopes in Surgical Therapy

Several potential surgical approaches have been considered in the treatment of refractory TGN. While MVD is performed to remove the neurovascular compression, percutaneous destructive procedures target the retrogasserian portion of the trigeminal nerve and GKRS damages the trigeminal nerve root with a concentrated dose of radiation. There are numerous studies on the surgical treatment for TGN [34], but, it is difficult to evaluate the quality of these published surgical reports [35].

Nerve Combing

Nerve combing (**internal neurolysis**) is a kind of surgical strategy that splits the branches of trigeminal nerve longitudinally using a special fiber knife based on preoperative pain locations and intraoperative findings. Jie and colleagues studied 60 patients of idiopathic TGN, 28 of whom had no visible NVC intraoperatively and 32 patients had presence of NVC. These patients had failed to respond to pharmacotherapy and underwent trigeminal nerve combing. All of them achieved good pain relief following nerve combing, but the relief rate was higher in patients without NVC than those with NVC [36].

Carbon-Dioxide (CO_2) Laser

Sessirisombat carried out a preliminary study to evaluate the results of CO_2 laser for the treatment of TGN. Thirty-six patients with drug-refractory TGN were enrolled to undergo peripheral nerve ablation with CO_2 laser using low-power defocused mode. The pain intensity was determined by numerical rating scales before and after operation. There was significant reduction in pain scores between pre-operation and 1 week, 1, 3, 6, and 12 months post-operation period. The author suggested neural ablation with CO_2 laser can be an alternative treatment for patients with TGN who do not respond to medical management and those who cannot tolerate/refuse to undergo intracranial procedure [37].

Neuromodulation

Several neuromodulation techniques have been tried as treatment options for pain refractory to conventional treatment, such as ***motor cortex stimulation (MCS)*** and ***deep brain stimulation (DBS)***. Studies have documented good results with MCS and DBS in TGN with 75–100% of patients achieving pain relief [38, 39]. Another alternative approach was suggested by Franzini et al. [41], who reported use of chronic posterior hypothalamus stimulation. In another study, patients suffering from refractory neuropathic trigeminal pain did not benefit from DBS, whereas patients with refractory TGN due to multiple sclerosis undergoing DBS at posterior hypothalamus, experienced a significant decrease in pain [42].

Repetitive Transcranial Magnetic Stimulation (rTMS) is a therapeutic method evaluates whether patients with TGN will respond to direct epidural cortical stimulation by measuring their response to an initial non-invasive cortical stimulation. In a study of patients with chronic intractable TGN with failed surgery, 58% experienced reduction in pain after receiving TMS [40]. Khedr et al., in another series of 24 patients, who were given rTMS to the motor cortex at 20 Hz daily for 5 days, pain rating was observed to be reduced by 45% [41].

There are limited number of studies on the long-term efficacy of neuromodulation, hence, it is difficult to evaluate its efficacy. However, these emerging techniques represent an opportunity in TGN treatment refractory to other treatments.

Conclusion

The treatment of TGN is a challenge for the pain physicians. Lack of a full comprehension of the complex pathogenesis is the key factor that produces unsatisfactory results to medical therapy. In the recent years a lot of progress has been made both in understanding the disease pathogenesis as well as surgical options along with improved neuroradiological interventions. Surgery has been presumed to be advantageous after the introduction of the endoscope and neuronavigation technologies. New drugs, such as botulinum neurotoxin, may be offered to these patients before surgery or to those who are unwilling to undergo surgery. Better definition of GKRS targets may improve the results of this technique. Neuromodulation represents another opportunity in refractory TGN patients, however, further studies may be required to elucidate its role with clarity.

References

1. Sindrup SH, Jensen TS. Pharmacotherapy of trigeminal neuralgia. Clin J Pain. 2002;18:22–7.
2. Cruccu G, Sommer C, Anand P, Attal N, Baron R, Garcia-Larrea L, et al. EFNS guidelines on neuropathic pain assessment: revised 2009. Eur J Neurol. 2010;17:1010–8.
3. Beydoun A. Clinical use of tricyclic anticonvulsants in painful neuropathies and bipolar disorders. Epilepsy Behav. 2002;3:S18–22.
4. Beydoun A. Safety and efficacy of oxcarbazepine: results of randomized, double-blind trials. Pharmacotherapy. 2000;20:152S–8S.
5. Liebel JT, Menger N, Langohr H. Oxcarbazepine in derBehandlung der Trigeminusneuralgie. Nervenheilkunde. 2001;20:461–5.
6. Montano N, Conforti G, Di Bonaventura R, Meglio M, Fernandez E, Papacci F. Advances in diagnosis and treatment of trigeminal neuralgia. Ther Clin Risk Manag. 2015;11:289–99.
7. Zakrzewska JM, Chaudhry Z, Nurmikko TJ, Patton DW, Mullens EL. Lamotrigine (Lamictal) in refractory trigeminal neuralgia: results from a double-blind placebo-controlled crossover trial. Pain. 1997;73:223–30.
8. Wiffen PJ, Derry S, Moore RA. Lamotrigine for acute and chronic pain. Cochrane Database Syst Rev. 2011;2:CD006044.
9. Fromm GH, Aumentado D, Terrence CF. A clinical and experimental investigation of the effects of tizanidine in trigeminal neuralgia. Pain. 1993;53:265–71.
10. Nurmikko TJ, Eldridge PR. Trigeminal neuralgia–pathophysiology, diagnosis and current treatment. Br J Anaesth. 2001;87:117–32.
11. Zakrzewska JM, Linskey ME. Trigeminal neuralgia. BMJ. 2014;348:g474.
12. Hu Y, Guan X, Fan L, Li M, Liao Y, Nie Z, Jin L. Therapeutic efficacy and safety of botulinum toxin type A in trigeminal neuralgia: a systematic review. J Headache Pain. 2013;14:72.
13. Cruccu G, Truini A. Refractory trigeminal neuralgia. Non-surgical treatment options. CNS Drugs. 2013;27:91–6.
14. Zakrzewska JM, Palmer J, Morisset V, Giblin GM, Obermann M, Ettlin D, et al., Study Investigators. Safety and efficacy of a Nav1.7 selective sodium channel blocker in patients with trigeminal neuralgia: a double-blind, placebo-controlled, randomised withdrawal phase 2A trial. Lancet Neurol. 2017;16:291–300.
15. Nurmikko TJ, Elderidge PR. Trigeminal neuralgia-pathophysiology, diagnosis and current treatment. Br J Anaesth. 2001;87:117–32.
16. Oturai AB, Jensen K, Erikson J, Marsden F. Neurosurgery for trigeminal neuralgia: comparison of alcohol block, neurectomy and radiofrequency coagulation. Clin J Pain. 1996;12:311–5.
17. Zakrzewska JM, Nally FF. The role of cryotherapy (cryoanalgesia) in the management of paroxysmal trigeminal neuralgia: a six-year experience. Br J Oral Maxillofac Surg. 1988;26:18–25.
18. Stefanoff V. Treatment of trigeminal neuralgia (TN) with local laser irradiation and laser puncture. Int J Oral Maxillofac Surg. 1990;19:379–80.
19. Samosiuk IZ, Kozhanova AK, Samosiuk NI. Physiopuncture therapy of trigeminal neuralgia. Vopr Kurortol Fizioter Lech Fiz Kult. 2000:29–32.
20. Scrivani SJ, Keith DA, Mathews ES, Kaban LB. Percutaneous stereotactic differential radiofrequency thermal rhizotomy for the treatment of trigeminal neuralgia. J Oral Maxillofac Surg. 1999;57:104–11.
21. Hakansson S. Trigeminal neuralgia treated by the injection into the trigeminal cistern. Neurosurgery. 1981;9:638–46.
22. Kouzounias K, Schechtmann G, Lind G, Winter J, Linderoth B. Factors that influence outcome of percutaneous balloon compression in the treatment of trigeminal neuralgia. Neurosurgery. 2010;67:925–34.
23. Abdennebi B, Mahfouf L, Nedjahi T. Long-term results of percutaneous compression of the gasserian ganglion in trigeminal neuralgia. Stereotact Funct Neurosurg. 1997;68:190–5.
24. Lichtor T, Mullan JF. A 10-year follow-up review of percutaneous micro-compression of the trigeminal ganglion. J Neurosurg. 1990;72:49–54.

25. Cruccu G, Gronseth G, Alksne J, Argoff C, Brainin M, Burchiel K, et al. AAN-EFNS guidelines on trigeminal neuralgia management. Eur J Neurol. 2008;15:1013–28.
26. Gu W, Zhao W. Microvascular decompression for recurrent trigeminal neuralgia. J Clin Neurosci. 2014;21:1549–53.
27. Broggi G, Ferroli P, Franzini A, Servello D, Dones I. Microvascular decompression for trigeminal neuralgia: comments on a series of 250 cases, including 10 patients with multiple sclerosis. J Neurol Neurosurg Psychiatry. 2000;68:59–64.
28. Oesman C, Mooij JJ. Long-term follow-up of microvascular decompression for trigeminal neuralgia. Skull Base. 2011;21:313–22.
29. Kondo A. Follow-up results of microvascular decompression in trigeminal neuralgia and hemifacial spasm. Neurosurgery. 1997;40:46–52.
30. Jafree DJ, Williams AC, Zakrzewska JM. Impact of pain and postoperative complications on patient-reported outcome measures 5 years after microvascular decompression or partial sensory rhizotomy for trigeminal neuralgia. Acta Neurochir. 2018;160:125–34.
31. Han JH, Kim DG, Chung HT, Paek SH, Kim YH, Kim CY, et al. Long-term outcome of gamma knife radiosurgery for treatment of typical trigeminal neuralgia. Int J Radiat Oncol Biol Phys. 2009;75:822–7.
32. Gronseth G, Cruccu G, Alksne J, Argoff C, Brainin M, Burchiel K, et al. Practice parameter: the diagnostic evaluation and treatment of trigeminal neuralgia (an evidence-based review): report of the Quality Standards Subcommittee of the American Academy of Neurology and the European Federation of Neurological Societies. Neurology. 2008;71:1183–90.
33. Zakrzewska JM, Lopez BC, Kim SE, Coakham HB. Patient reports of satisfaction after microvascular decompression and partial sensory rhizotomy for trigeminal neuralgia. Neurosurgery. 2005;56:1304–11.
34. Tatli M, Satici O, Kanpolat Y, Sindou M. Various surgical modalities for trigeminal neuralgia: literature study of respective long-term outcomes. Acta Neurochir. 2008;150:243–55.
35. Akram H, Mirza B, Kitchen N, Zakrzewska JM. Proposal for evaluating the quality of reports of surgical interventions in the treatment of trigeminal neuralgia: the surgical trigeminal neuralgia score. Neurosurg Focus. 2013;35:E3.
36. Jie H, Xuanchen Z, Deheng L, Kun G, Fengyang X, Xiang C, et al. The long-term outcome of nerve combing for trigeminal neuralgia. Acta Neurochir. 2013;155:1703–8.
37. Sessirisombat S. Carbon-dioxide laser in the treatment of trigeminal neuralgia: a preliminary study. J Interdiscipl Med Dent Sci. 2017;5:1–4.
38. Fontaine D, Hamani C, Lozano A. Efficacy and safety of motor cortex stimulation for chronic neuropathic pain: critical review of the literature. J Neurosurg. 2009;110:251–6.
39. Buchanan RJ, Darrow D, Monsivais D, Nadasdy Z, Gjini K. Motor cortex stimulation for neuropathic pain syndromes: a case series experience. Neuroreport. 2014;25:715–7.
40. Lefaucheur JP, Drouot X, Menard-Lefaucheur I, Zerah F, Bendib B, Cesaro P, et al. Neurogenic pain relief by repetitive transcranial magnetic cortical stimulation depends on the origin and the site of pain. J Neurol Neurosurg Psychiatry. 2004;75:612–6.
41. Khedr EM, Kotb H, Kamel NF, Ahmed MA, Sadek R, Rothwell JC. Long lasting antalgic effects of daily sessions of repetitive transcranial magnetic stimulation in central and peripheral neuropathic pain. J Neurol Neurosurg Psychiatry. 2005;76:833–8.

MIX
Papier aus verantwortungsvollen Quellen
Paper from responsible sources
FSC® C105338

If you have any concerns about our products,
you can contact us on
ProductSafety@springernature.com

In case Publisher is established outside the EU,
the EU authorized representative is:
Springer Nature Customer Service Center GmbH
Europaplatz 3, 69115 Heidelberg, Germany

Printed by Libri Plureos GmbH
in Hamburg, Germany